MW01283578

What Others Are Saying About *Proud But Never Satisfied*

Hospitals are America's most complex organizations and often the most resistant to innovation. This book uniquely lays out the transformation of The University of Kansas Hospital—now The University of Kansas Health System—into one of the best healthcare providers in the country. But it does more than that. It also shows leaders and engaged employees of any organization under stress how to identify and focus on the right outcome metrics, how to improve underperforming teams by linking them to top-performing groups, how to structure and support innovation across different fields or disciplines, and ultimately how to respond to a crisis like COVID-19 with effective communication, empathy, and action—in effect, how to build and sustain a culture of organizational innovation and success.

—Arthur Daemmrich, Director, Smithsonian Lemelson Center for the Study of Invention and Innovation

KU Health System is an incredible turnaround story—and one I'm glad we supported financially many years ago. They turned adversity into advantage. That's real transformation, and this book explains how to do that in one of the toughest businesses there is today: healthcare.

—Philip F. Anschutz

This is so cool, humble, poignant, moving, inspiring, insightful, and worthy. *Proud But Never Satisfied* is something that leaders in healthcare will read.

—Mike Rona, Partner, Moss Adams; Former President, Virginia Mason Medical Center

I have read many leadership books and witnessed many business transformations. The lessons Tammy and Bob share about The University of Kansas Health System are among the best—empowering teamwork, collaboration, and valuing the important role everyone has to play. Engaging the heart of every nurse, every doctor, and every support staff member is at the root of their success. These lessons are best taught in practice. At The University of Kansas Health System, the results speak for themselves.

—David Dillon, Retired Chairman and CEO, The Kroger Co.

From two of the most successful healthcare leaders in America comes the seminal book on healthcare transformation.

Page and Peterman argue convincingly that transformation begins with attitude. Duty, strategy, and technology all play their part, but it starts with a culture that supports the "proud but never satisfied" mindset. This is the seminal book on that approach, and how it turned one of America's lowest-rated hospitals into one of its greatest.

—Greg Graves, Former CEO, Burns & McDonnell Engineering; Author of *Create Amazing*

It's no surprise that back when TUKHS had the worst patient satisfaction in the nation, it *also* had astronomical employee turnover. Nor is it surprising that today, when it's consistently ranked as one of America's best hospitals, it has some of the lowest turnover. Employee engagement always goes hand-in-hand with performance. *Proud But Never Satisfied* is a success story on many fronts. But from my viewpoint, it's a treatise on what's possible when you can get team members at all levels to buy into a bold vision and throw their hearts and souls into making it happen. In an age where a high-engagement culture is mandatory for survival, this blueprint for transformation can bring us all hope.

—Craig Deao, MHA; Author of *The E-Factor: How Engaged Patients, Clinicians, Leaders, and Employees Will Transform Healthcare*

One thing I know is that leadership begins and ends with putting others first. When The University of Kansas Hospital made patients the priority—actually based their business model on a people-first culture—that was leadership at its finest. And it certainly paid off, as this book explains. There are lessons here, not just for healthcare but for humanity.

—Dayton Moore, General Manager, Kansas City Royals; Author of *More Than a Season*

What really strikes me about this story is not simply the successful transformation—but how The University of Kansas Health System sustained a high level of success over time by constantly challenging themselves to improve. *Proud But Never Satisfied* is more than the title of Page and Peterman's book; it is a mantra for their entire organization.

—Clark Hunt, Chairman and CEO, Kansas City Chiefs

To me, some of the most fascinating parts of this book center on how The University of Kansas Health System responded to COVID-19. Not only did they take a leadership role in helping educate and support the community, they instantly got to work addressing the emotional, psychological, and practical needs of their employees. No wonder this hospital is widely known as a great place to work! They clearly see that patient experience and employee experience are intertwined. This current crisis surely isn't our last—and it's the organizations that deliberately seek to create cultures of resilience that will be the winners.

—Gary R. Simonds, MD, MHCDS; Coauthor of *Thriving in Healthcare: A Positive Approach to Reclaim Balance and Avoid Burnout in Your Busy Life* and *The Thriving Physician: How to Avoid Burnout by Choosing Resilience Throughout Your Medical Career*

My specialty is helping physicians and other providers build resilience so they can avoid burnout and thrive in high-stress conditions. But individual resilience doesn't spring up in a vacuum. Its presence is inseparable from how leaders lead, and how fervently an organization engages employees and supports their well-being. *Proud But Never Satisfied* shines a light on how The University of Kansas Health System created a strong, agile culture.

Many of their tactics—from great training to reward and recognition to storytelling that builds passion and purpose—plant the seeds of resilience in their people. A compelling book, and one we all need in today's environment.

—Wayne M. Sotile, PhD; Coauthor of *Thriving in Healthcare: A Positive Approach to Reclaim Balance and Avoid Burnout in Your Busy Life* and *The Thriving Physician: How to Avoid Burnout by Choosing Resilience Throughout Your Medical Career*

Proud But Never Satisfied

Ten Transformative Actions for Healthcare Systems

THE UNIVERSITY OF KANSAS HEALTH SYSTEM

Bob Page and Tammy Peterman

with Leeanne Seaver

Huron Consulting Services, LLC

Published by:
Huron Consulting Services, LLC
550 W. Van Buren Street
Chicago, IL 60607
Phone: (312) 583-8700
www.huronconsultinggroup.com

ISBN: 978-1-62218-111-7

Library of Congress Control Number: 2020945220

This book was published by Huron Consulting Services, LLC, a global consultancy that collaborates with clients to drive strategic growth, ignite innovation, and navigate constant change.

The stories in this book are true. However, some names and identifying details have been changed to protect the privacy of all concerned. Any reference in this publication to any person or organization; activities, products, or services related to any named person or organization; or any political party, platform, or candidate, do not constitute or imply the endorsement, recommendation, or favoring of Huron, its affiliates, or any employees or contractors acting on their behalf.

Printed in the United States of America

To those who came before us, to those with whom we have had the honor and privilege to work side by side, and to those who will follow us and keep this journey alive well into the future, this book is for you.

Table of Contents

Foreword

I have been watching The University of Kansas Health System for almost two decades now—since it was a very sick hospital in desperate need of a lifeline. It found one by jumping *off* the bandwagon of how healthcare usually works in this country. This gutsy group decided to challenge the status quo with a unique approach to saving lives, including its own.

Today, The University of Kansas Health System is recognized among the top academic hospitals in the country and has been nationally ranked for more than a decade as one of the best hospitals in America by *U.S. News & World Report*.[1] Those remarkable achievements and more belong to this extraordinary, world-class hospital in the heartland—the same one that had the lowest patient satisfaction ranking in the nation in the '90s.

The University of Kansas Health System saved itself by effectively transforming its vision and mission into a business model. *Proud But Never Satisfied* tells how they pulled that off by ignoring a lot of the old adages—by finding success without selling their soul. Here are those lessons. Here are the business model and evidence-based outcomes. And here are stories of the culture and community that made this happen. It happened because The University of Kansas Hospital made a brave, unorthodox decision two decades ago that changed its destiny.

Today, The University of Kansas Health System continues to advance healthcare, not only in the heart of America, but across our country.

—Quint Studer,
Founder, Studer Group

Preface

Imagine you have just been appointed the CEO of an organization with the following challenges:

- You have the worst customer satisfaction scores in your industry.
- You are unable to accurately measure the quality of the service you provide.
- Your staff turnover is 33 percent annually.
- Your recent employee opinion survey results indicate your employees…
    - would not recommend your organization as a place to work
    - would not recommend your product
    - are not proud to work at your organization
- Your volumes are declining despite the growth in your industry's market.
- You have no money.

Where do you start? *No margin = no mission*, so the focus must clearly be on finances, right?

Maybe not.

Imagine risking everything on a philosophical belief instead of a proven business model.

What if people *came first—starting with patients but including staff—rather than growing market share and improving bottom-line performance?*

How can the right culture transform your organization from the lowest to among the highest performers nationwide?

What does it take to develop, operationalize, and sustain that? How does that stand up through a pandemic?

Proud But Never Satisfied is for everyone who's asked us how we answered those questions at The University of Kansas Health System—and also for those who didn't know to ask but desperately need the answer themselves. Here are the lessons we've learned along the way and ten transformative actions that can work for your organization, too.

—Bob Page and Tammy Peterman

What's in a Name?

The University of Kansas Health System has been the official name of this comprehensive academic medical center since 2016-17, although that title was being used as early as 2012. That name represents the evolution of an organization that was first established in 1906 as The University of Kansas Hospital—the clinical arm of The University of Kansas School of Medicine.

During its first 92 years of operation, KU Hospital (KUH) was referred to and recognized by many names, including KU Med/KU Medical Center. With its independence from the state system in 1998, its official name became The University of Kansas Hospital Authority. People have used the name they were most familiar with over the years…it can be confusing.

Throughout this book, KU Health System's varying names are used accurately in context to the timeline of the organization. For example, The University of Kansas Hospital (KUH) references things that happened before 2012, or things that happen specifically at the main campus. Since 2012, The University of Kansas Health System or TUKHS is used to encompass not only the broader scope of practice but the larger footprint that includes affiliated hospitals statewide.

Acknowledgments

In orientation, we tell our new employees they have two choices. They can sit back and read the book about what has been learned on our journey, or they can roll up their sleeves and help us write the story. *Proud But Never Satisfied* is dedicated to the thousands of individuals who contributed a paragraph, page, or chapter in this ongoing story of transformation.

Thanks to Quint Studer, for providing guidance and counsel since our paths first crossed in 1999 as we began our transformation. Your coaching and support were key to helping us kick off our journey. We hope we made you proud (but not satisfied).

Thank you, Irene Thompson, for setting the table with your visionary leadership and ability to put together a team that withstood the test of time. To this day, your strategic decisions continue to benefit our health system. And, most of all, thank you for believing in us.

To the leaders of the University of Kansas, The University of Kansas Medical Center, and the legislators who helped give form to The University of Kansas Hospital Authority, none of this would have been possible without your courage and commitment to change the governance structure of our hospital. The legislation you helped create and pass changed the face of our organization in ways yet to be discovered.

To our staff—those who were here from the beginning and those who have joined over the years because they believed in what was happening here and wanted to make a difference—you have our deepest thanks. None of what we share in this book would have been possible without your commitment, your passion, and your hard work. We are a better place for patient care, a better place to work, and a better resource for our community because of you.

To our physicians: So many of you have been with us since this journey began in the late '90s, and hundreds more have joined us over the years. You have been amazing partners in the work we have undertaken to build a nationally recognized academic medical center. You've made numerous leaps of faith that weren't easy, but necessary in the creation of this health system, not the least of which was clinical integration. We are a better place because of you.

To those who have supported our journey with your financial backing, so much of what we have accomplished has happened because of your belief in us, your support of our organization, and your advocacy for this health system. Your generosity has rippled through and beyond the organization in ways you may not know. Your recognition of what the health system is doing has given energy and pride to our team and sent a message to others in the community that the amazing work being done here is worthy of support.

To our partners within The University of Kansas Medical Center who were part of this journey since the beginning—we are two sides of the same coin, working together to advance education, research, and patient care. The pandemic has brought us to new levels of collaboration and partnership in support of our staff, the people in our community, and the citizens across the state. We are better together and thankful for the ongoing gift of your friendship, collaboration, and strategic partnership.

To those who have served and currently serve on our board of directors, your support, advice, friendship, and firm counsel have played a major role in getting us to where we are today. You have invested your knowledge, your passion, your time, and your reputation in helping us grow as an organization and advance in the eyes of the community. You have always been there to celebrate our team, promote us throughout the community, and tell our story wherever possible. We are forever in your debt.

Thanks to our families. Your support, love, encouragement, and belief in what we are doing truly made our contributions possible. You have walked this journey with us and been instrumental in what has been accomplished. Your willingness to give us the time to do this work has freed our hearts and minds to help our health system achieve more than was ever thought possible. We will be forever grateful for the sacrifices you have made throughout the years.

Thanks to Leeanne Seaver, who taught us how to write a book, how to find the nuggets to share, and how to set deadlines so this book would finally become a reality. Thanks for knowing how to apply pressure appropriately and ease up when necessary. Your belief in our story was not only validating but inspirational. You have been a joy to work with and we will be forever grateful for your time, commitment, skills, and friendship.

And finally, to Terry Rusconi, we couldn't have done this without you. You have been with us since the beginning. We have been partners throughout this journey. We have learned from each other, depended on each other, and lived through the highs and lows together. To complete this book during a pandemic is a tribute to your amazing recall, your dedication and commitment to our organization, your ability to help us capture the essence of any situation, and your remarkable character. Thank you.

—Bob Page and Tammy Peterman

So many amazing people shared their experiences and expertise to help me get this remarkable story right. I am so thankful to each of you who will recognize yourselves in these chapters.

In particular, Jill Chadwick, Greg Graves, Chris Ruder, Becky Pilarz, Alex Welborn, Kathryn Verlin, Bob Honse, Gigi Siers, Arthur Daemmrich, Tori Butler, and William Reed (posthumously): Thank you for loving this institution enough to field a call from me at 11:30 p.m. on a Saturday night, if necessary (true story).

Terry, thank you for "The Rusconi Effect." You are the patron of TUKHS culture, and your influence has improved every page.

Finally, I am inexpressibly grateful to Bob Page and Tammy Peterman for trusting me. This has always been more than a commission; it's been an honor and privilege to write with you. Your leadership has operationalized a culture that truly puts people first. Many doubt that's really possible in healthcare today.

Well, here's what I know…every day you write the book.

—Leeanne Seaver

CHAPTER ONE

Admit It

You can't change what you refuse to confront.
—Anonymous

Just before midnight on October 1, 2018, a group gathered in the hospital lobby. News crews were setting up cameras as the crowd of senior executives, current staff plus former hospital employees, civic leaders, dignitaries, and community members grew to nearly 100.

At exactly 12:00 a.m., solemnity fell over the scene, and senior executives Bob Page and Tammy Peterman approached the podium. What they were about to say would have been hard to imagine 20 years earlier, on that same day in 1998. That was the point of the gathering, and the point of this book. Some had dared to imagine it, and then actually made it happen, so there was a lot to be said about The University of Kansas Health System (TUKHS) on this night.

Some had dared to imagine it, and then actually made it happen.

"Thank you for coming out at this hour," Page said into the mic. "This is about bringing our past and our present together." Those in the crowd proudly holding paddle-signs printed with "20 Years" knew the story—especially how it came dangerously close to never being told.

Where We've Been Is Not Where We Are Now

When Bob Page first arrived at The University of Kansas Hospital in October 1996, no one seemed to be expecting him. There was some uncertainty as to who he was and where his office should be. In the midst of the confusion, Page was surprised by a familiar face.

"I walked into the executive office, and my former boss, who had been CEO of Jewish Hospital in St. Louis, was sitting in a chair," recalled Page. "I said, 'Wayne, what are you doing here?' He said, 'I am working for a consulting firm.' I said, 'Oh, good. What are you working on?' He answered, 'Well, I am helping your hospital.' I said, 'With what?' He said, 'To see if it can survive.'"

That was Day One. Over the next few weeks, Page, a Price Waterhouse alum and former director of audit services at BJC HealthCare in St. Louis, gained a sense of what he was up against. As the first vice president of organizational improvement, a new department of which he was the only member, Page was tasked with raising the performance bar. But first there would be the problem of finding it. There were no dashboards or performance data—serious red flags indicative of the hospital's broader dilemma.

"It occurred to me that I hadn't really done my homework before taking the job," Page admitted, adding that he was hardly the only one unaware. "Most of the people in this hospital didn't even realize what kind of trouble we were in."

That was about to change dramatically.

Admittedly, the healthcare industry itself had no standardized quantifiable measures of quality in the late 20th century. The introduction of the concept from Carey and Lloyd's groundbreaking *Measuring Quality Improvement in Healthcare* came in the mid-'90s.[1] To the extent that anyone was applying quality measures to hospital performance, they were adapting models from the automotive industry.[2] As such, The University of Kansas Hospital didn't have readily available data reflecting its dire straits—but the signs were undeniable.

To the extent that anyone was applying quality measures to hospital performance in the '90s, they were adapting models from the automotive industry.

Across vast floors of the 850,000-square-foot main campus were vacant units and empty beds.

"There were entire floors shut down," said Dr. Bruce Toby, who had come to KU Hospital (KUH) in 1991.

Dr. Toby, who would go on to become chair of orthopedic surgery at The University of Kansas Medical Center, reported the census was less than half the capacity.

"There were so few patients they could consolidate them into a few floors," he recalled. "There would be more doctors and students on rounds than they would have patients. There wasn't a whole lot to do all the time. They couldn't get equipment or normal supplies in the OR, because they had to go through the state system. They had to get approval from legislators in Topeka. I'd never seen anything like it. It was absolutely bizarre."[3]

Patient volume had been dropping for decades—up to 5 percent annually in spite of robust market growth. Discharges bottomed out at 13,000 in 1998—down from 21,281 in 1971.[4] And the mortality index showed that more patients died than would be expected based upon their condition.

The problem of staff turnover cost KUH a third of its workforce annually. Employees wouldn't recommend it for care or employment to their own family members. Between 1995 and '98, its already-ailing reputation was hard-hit by two major PR disasters: a debacle that shut down its heart transplant program and a newborn kidnapping.

Topping the long list of organizational ills in the mid-'90s was this dubious record: The hospital had the lowest patient satisfaction rank in the nation at a humiliating 5th percentile.

Topping the long list of organizational ills in the mid-'90s was this dubious record: The hospital had the lowest patient satisfaction rank in the nation at a humiliating 5th percentile.[5] And one unrelenting reality kept KUH in its tailspin: The hospital had no money. Indeed, it was the institution that patients went to when they had no insurance or money to pay for their care, so funding was a long-standing problem.

For 92 years—since The University of Kansas Hospital began its operation as the clinical arm of The University of Kansas Medical School—every dollar earned at the end of the year went back to the academic enterprise, leaving the hospital with no funds for improvements, repairs, or competitive hiring. As a business model, it was unsustainable, but as a state agency, it was just business as usual.

"At that time, I didn't know how poorly the organization was doing," recalled Tammy Peterman, RN, who would go on to become president of the Kansas City Division, executive vice president, and COO/CNO of The University of Kansas Health System. "If the performance figures were there, they weren't shared widely—if at all."

LEADERSHIP LESSON:

We had to admit it to ourselves as an organization:
We had a very serious problem.

The issue of the hospital's survival had been officially raised by Irene Thompson (then Cumming). Thompson was newly appointed as chief executive officer in April 1996. She was a former Price Waterhouse partner and the chief financial officer of a major health system in Pennsylvania before starting at KU Hospital as CFO in 1994. Thompson was promoted to COO, then functioned as an unofficial/acting CEO. After the beleaguered CEO finally resigned in the midst of the heart transplant scandal in '96, Thompson stepped into her new role and took stock.

"My impression of the hospital was that it was under-capitalized," she said. "My impression of the people was that they were really dedicated, but without an organization or management that would enable them to function at their highest levels. There were many people with authority but no accountability."[6]

There were many people with authority but no accountability.

The hospital's challenges on every front were weighted with a fiscal urgency that was intensifying. By 1996, in-patient care volume was 30 percent lower than it had been in 1975.[7] The roof leaked, and the equipment was antiquated. Neither minor repairs nor major capital improvements could be addressed for lack of funds. Technologies were out of date, and facilities were in serious decline.

Needless to say, the hospital was in financial trouble. The bottom line approached negative, and it was clear something had to be done. Cost-cutting on bare bones wasn't a long-term solution, but immediate strategies for inventory control were put in place. Vacant positions went unfilled. This tightened the budget, if painfully, and bought its new CEO some time. But it wasn't going to save the hospital.

"We couldn't cut ourselves to growth," Thompson said.

LEADERSHIP LESSON:

Cost-cutting on bare bones is not a long-term solution. Layoffs, inventory control, and culling through attrition may buy some time, but, as the saying goes, you can't shrink your way to greatness.

What If There Were No Hospital?

It was clear to Thompson, Page, and executive leadership that the status quo needed to change, but not at the cost of what was still working. In spite of it all, The University of Kansas Hospital still had a purpose that was deeply rooted in the community. Its origins stretch back to 1905, when Dr. Simeon Bell gave $50,000 and 35 acres at "Goat Hill" just southwest of downtown Kansas City to establish a much-needed hospital for The University of Kansas School of Medicine. Today, an imprint of Bell's words on the walls encircles the hospital's main foyer. "This shall be a place where the people of Kansas and areas surrounding may enjoy the best medical care available anywhere."

Market Changes Produce Ill Effects for Academic Medical Centers

In the early 1990s, shifts in market forces began to adversely affect academic hospitals across the country. First, full implementation of the diagnosis related group (DRG) system by Medicare squeezed annual growth in government payments that previously compensated academic hospitals for their inefficient cost structures that included staffing by interns and residents alongside senior physicians. Second, new restrictions were put on Medicaid payments that compensated hospitals for charity care. Third, managed care fostered narrow network alliances between insurers and care providers and reduced referrals to academic centers from community hospitals and local physicians. Nationally, over 50 million Americans were insured by health maintenance organizations (HMOs) in 1995. Locally, the Kansas City market was "characterized by provider consolidation, declining admissions, and deep payment discounts." Fourth, competitors of the KU Hospital consolidated during the early 1990s, with Research Medical Center (owned by Health Midwest), St. Luke's, and Shawnee Mission emerging as market leaders. Revenues shrank as admissions to the KU Hospital declined by 8.4 percent between 1993 and 1996. Faculty at KU Med began to struggle to find cases needed to teach students and residents. In intensive care, admissions shrank to as few as four patients daily.[8]
—Arthur Daemmrich, PhD

There had been years of progress and accomplishment, but since the comparatively robust '70s, the slow deterioration of KU Hospital had been widely seen and felt. Changes in the healthcare industry and the functional limitations of the hospital's governance system were causal, and the aforementioned PR scandals in the mid-'90s were certainly catalytic.

Then-COO Jon Jackson acknowledged, "Bureaucracy led to people not stepping forward and doing things they needed to do and to poor decision-making about sale versus retained-ownership of assets of the organization. Scandal led to loss of public trust and loss of income."[9]

It was a perfect storm.

"We had to turn the *Titanic* around," Bob Page said.

That would be the herculean task of leadership. With disarming frankness, Thompson recruited her former colleagues Scott Glasrud and Chris Hansen. As the new chief financial officer, Glasrud got started on the balance sheet and creating financial systems for over 2,000 employees.[10] Hansen, who would go on to become senior vice president for ambulatory services and chief information officer, went to work on expanding the outpatient footprint for primary care around the community.

The work was daunting; this would not be business as usual.

"Irene said right off the bat that it was a turnaround situation and that she was looking for somebody she could really partner with," Glasrud recalled.

This would not be business as usual.

Confidence in Thompson was part of the draw. In fact, Bob Page had used his Price Waterhouse connections to get the interview with her that secured his new position at KU Hospital. He joined the brain trust that made the next steps possible, acknowledging, "One of the things I really respected about Irene was that she knew how to put a team together. Then she knew to give us as much rope as we could handle and let us go."

LEADERSHIP LESSON:

Get the right people on the team, give them as much rope as they can handle, and then let go.

Heralding the hands-on approach that would eventually lead to his promotion to CEO and president of the hospital by 2007, Page dove in deep. He was less interested in the financial figures than the variability in care and how that could be improved and standardized.

"What if we could all perform at a certain level; what would that do for the hospital?" he said. "I just started asking a bunch of questions to find out what we were benchmarking against."

There was nothing automated to work from, so finally he "found the green bar reports that we used to print off in long runs," Page recalled. "So I got those reports, and I found myself with a pencil, piece of paper, and calculator. That's how I got started. I was just looking at stuff. Quite frankly, it took a long time."

But a data story was emerging.

Page was less interested in the financial figures than the variability in care and how that could be improved and standardized.

Thompson took on the administrative constraints on the hospital's operations and "an organizational culture that consisted of workarounds and attention to hierarchy rather than a focus on patients."[11] To inform and objectify a broader view, she proposed hiring independent consultants, the Lash Group, to analyze the situation and help her "figure out how to keep the place afloat."

Robert Hemenway, chancellor of the University of Kansas, was receptive to the idea.

"Fortunately, I had Chancellor Hemenway to work with," Thompson said. "He was extremely reasonable. He would listen to everyone. He would take the time to learn and then make a decision. And he didn't make political decisions, which was uncommon in a state university setting."

The Lash Report

By November 1996, the consultants presented their findings in the "Lash Report." It revealed the chest-tightening news that the hospital was on course to cost the state of Kansas millions annually.

"If we didn't change anything, it was projected we would have to put at least $20 million a year of the State General Fund into the hospital beginning in 2000," former State

Representative Kenny Wilk recalled. "Actually, none of us believed that. We figured we'd have to start putting money in sooner. We also assumed it would have to be more than $20 million a year."[12]

Of six possible scenarios detailed in the Lash Report,[13] the discussions whittled the options down to three:

1. Sell it
2. Close it
3. Make it a public authority

The Lash Group's recommendation was for the third option, specifically, to establish the hospital as a public authority with its own board of directors and governance that could legally function autonomously within the state system. With this new freedom, the hospital could operate more like an independent business—obtaining funding for long-term strategic growth, paying market-based wages rather than what the state deemed appropriate, and creating a culture focused on what could be done rather than regularly being told why things couldn't be done.

This would require a change in state law—a process that wasn't without risk as legislators could amend the proposed bill, adding provisions impacting how the hospital would operate. The political climate in Kansas was conservative in 1997. (Then-Governor Bill Graves pointed out the majority were "all for privatization. If you put the word 'privatization' into anything, you'd have about two-thirds of the legislature behind you.")[14]

It took two sessions to pull it off, with Hemenway getting much-deserved credit for the successful lobby that would result in the passage of Senate Bill 373 in February 1998.

"That's how it developed," Thompson said. "I was pleased that there was support to do something different with the hospital. I was pleased there was a solution that gave us ownership and the freedom to operate as a business."

The Burning Platform

To survive, The University of Kansas Hospital had to overcome obstacles on three fronts: politics, business, and medicine. While the first was being addressed legislatively,

Thompson and Bob Page were undertaking an internal campaign to reality-check staff on the second and third, and prepare them for the changes to come. Getting people to admit there was a problem was the first step. The operational dysfunction had gone on for so long it was considered normal, and that attitude lowered the bar every year.

"*Tension for change* is a management concept that says there must be a compelling force pushing an organization in a new direction," Page explained. "To create that tension, we had to establish the 'burning platform' so our own people could see what was really going on."[15]

LEADERSHIP LESSON:

There must be a compelling force pushing an organization in a new direction. We had to establish the "burning platform" so our own people could see what was really going on.

In December 1997, Irene Thompson launched a series of town hall meetings to educate staff on the hospital's current level of performance. The news was grim and hard to hear, but necessary.

Terry Rusconi, the newly hired director of organizational development, said, "Basically, Irene took the gloves off and told people just how much improvement we needed to make. The staff had never heard that. They didn't know that our patient satisfaction was so low or that all the other indicators were not where they needed to be. It really frightened a lot of people."

The platform was ignited.

The news was grim. It was hard to hear, but it was necessary.

It was an extremely vulnerable situation, but KUH had a powerful asset: the staff itself. Page knew "these people came here to take care of patients. That's why they went into healthcare."

There was strong alignment to purpose, but as Rusconi saw it, "The biggest obstacle was that employees had been hammered down by the state system for so long they didn't trust that they could make the changes that were needed. They had tried to make things better but were limited by the mentality that was part of the state's system at the time."

Now big changes were in the offing, and executive leadership was banking on a major course correction that would require all hands on deck.

LEADERSHIP LESSON:

We needed to let people know what our path to success was going to be.

Acknowledging the magnitude of the problem was a start, but it was crucial not to get stuck in the stage of problem admiration.

"There's risk in putting it all out there if there's not a plan to do something about it—just talking about it isn't enough," Rusconi said. "One of the things we learned was we needed to let people know what our path to success was going to be."[16]

Leadership had to make change possible, both functionally and psychologically. It had to articulate a vision that would inspire everyone to take the first steps to:

- Commit in spite of the risks
- Collaborate in unprecedented ways
- Create mechanisms to support the goal

Keeping the hospital doors open was the goal, but Bob Page admitted, "I got hung up on the idea that if you're going to set a goal, then set it as high as you possibly can."

Achieving that goal would begin with incremental steps that reinforced and validated progress along the way.

"It didn't happen overnight, which was hard for me—a Type-A personality," said Page. "But gradually we had to 'right-size' our thinking. We set the goal high, then started climbing. And we decided to benchmark ourselves against the best."

LEADERSHIP LESSON:

Set your goal as high as you possibly can but acknowledge incremental progress as you climb. It's important to validate achievement so everyone feels vested in a shared vision, not overwhelmed by it.

The Tension for Change

On October 1, 1998, The University of Kansas Hospital would officially cut the cord from the state system—marking the end of state subsidies.

"If we didn't separate, we couldn't succeed," Thompson explained.

During the town hall meetings, Thompson made it clear there was a need to progress at a different speed from ever before. Success was about actual results—not on perpetual analysis or theoretical review. Everyone was going to be accountable for deliverables—starting with leadership—and every process had to support outcomes. The tension for change had become the fuel to get up and go, but there was still the problem of the vehicle itself.

LEADERSHIP LESSON:

Success is about actual results—not perpetual analysis or theoretical review.

The newly independent hospital had no cash or accounting system, and no personnel or retirement system. Approximately 2,200 employees had to be exited from the state system—their retirement and healthcare programs transferred to the new entity that had no structures in place yet. Administrative policies and procedures for 18 different management and billing entities—one for each of the medical specialties on the joint campus—had to be operationalized.

Agreement with the Kansas University Physicians, Inc. (KUPI) group had to be reached so there would be a specific contract in place for physician services at the hospital. Then there were leases, subleases, and academic affiliation agreements to be negotiated with the medical school, as well as ownership of shared buildings on the campus to be divvied up.

Whether it was the reality of losing cash flow from the hospital's clinical operation or losing control of the hospital in general, The University of Kansas School of Medicine (i.e., KUMC: The University of Kansas Medical Center) was now feeling the strain of losing its clinical enterprise. Things came to a head once the closing agreements had to be signed.

Thompson remembered her anxiety at that meeting.

"I was rushing to the closing and I was a few minutes late," she recalled. "I was very concerned about that because, having been in many closings from tax exempt bond issues, I knew that we would have sets of documents all over the table and people all around the conference room. I was the one signing and I was embarrassed to be five minutes late.

"I ran into the conference room and there was Frank Ross, our attorney, on the phone all by himself talking to the Board of Regents' attorney saying, 'What do you mean you can't come?'" Thompson continued. "The Board of Regents' attorney said, 'I'm too busy today to come.' No one from the university came."

Thompson managed to track down Chancellor Hemenway in Washington, DC, and alert him to the situation. She didn't hear back from him directly, but at 5:00 p.m., representatives for the university came and mulled over the paperwork for several hours.

That was all the cash we had. It was enough money to cover payroll and operations for 30 days.

"They finally handed me a check at midnight," Thompson said. "Not even a wire transfer, but a check for $23.5 million. That was the cash. That was all the cash we had and we were off."

It was roughly enough money to cover payroll and operations for 30 days.

The Hail Mary Pass

The hard work of getting the bill passed was now behind them. "It was considered a 'Hail Mary pass,'" Kenny Wilk admitted. "The legislature didn't know if a public authority governance model would work, but everyone knew something had to happen. It was a gutsy move. If it failed, we were done."

The enabling legislation was now in place, but the harder work of implementation was still ahead.

> By creating The Kansas Hospital Authority, the state legislators did something really great in Topeka. They created this entity that was a component of state government and then by statute, they exempted it from just about every state law—the red tape that applies elsewhere in government but doesn't apply here, and shouldn't. This isn't an agency of the state that taxes or that regulates a business. It's not in the same vein, and they recognized that.[17]
> —Frank Ross, Attorney

The oversight and governance of The University of Kansas Hospital was spelled out in a section of the statute that had been innovatively crafted. No longer subject to the Kansas Board of Regents, the new authority provided for a 14-member hospital board of directors. Governor Graves appointed the first board, composed of six insiders and eight independent members, in 1998.

Bob Honse of Lawrence, Kansas, was one of those "outsiders" who joined the board in 2000. Honse was the president and CEO of Farmland Industries, one of the nation's largest agricultural cooperatives.

He was strongly recruited because "the governor basically wanted eight businesspeople—most of whom had no medical background," Honse recalled. "The idea was, 'If this were your business, what would you do?'"

And there was a lot to do—quickly.

"We used to jokingly say that long-term planning was that we anticipated coming back next month for a board meeting," said Honse.

If this were your business, what would you do?

What Honse and the other new board members did was apply corporate acumen to the hospital operation. No longer tied exclusively to the education and research agenda of the university, it was clear to the board their "product" was—without compromise—patient care.

"My hesitation about coming on the board was not the time commitment but where would I go if got sick," said Honse. "Did I have to come to this hospital? Because in 2000, this was not the hospital in town a person would want to go to. That was universally known. So that was my struggle."[18]

Honse's fears would be laid to rest over the course of his tenure on the board. He would need several surgeries and treatment for cancer. All were successful.

"Yes, I not only gained confidence, but the whole community gained confidence," Honse reflected. "Today, I refer everyone I know to KU Health System. It's the only place my wife and I go."

After serving as board chair the first year, Chancellor Hemenway stepped aside for George Farha. Farha had come to America from Lebanon as a young man to study medicine. He settled in Wichita, where he married and started a successful surgical practice in the late '50s. A consummate patient advocate, Dr. Farha had a terrific grasp of healthcare's academic and clinical aspects. Revered on the university side and by the hospital, he was the ideal choice for board chair in 1999.

LEADERSHIP LESSON:

Patients don't care how much you know until they know how much you care.

Meanwhile, Tammy Peterman had just accepted Bob Page's offer to join the Organizational Improvement Department.

"Dr. Farha always said, 'Put the patient first in everything you do,'" she stated. "The patient is the reason we are in business. Without the patient, we have no business.'"

His philosophy was empowered by his oft-repeated mantra: *Patients don't care how much you know until they know how much you care.*

As The University of Kansas Hospital Authority found its legs, Farha's patient-first philosophy provided the marching orders. Along that journey, The University of Kansas Hospital began transitioning to its new name, The University of Kansas Health System (TUKHS), in 2012—a name change that represented the new identity that emerged through the transformation.

That transformation focused on employee engagement and all key measures important to patient care and outcomes. It was calibrated with a goal Bob Page had articulated with his characteristic chutzpah back in 1999.

"Yeah, he made a bold, bold statement, very bold," Irene Thompson recalled, smiling. "I remember it wasn't my idea. Bob came into my office and said, 'So why don't we say we're going to be number one in the country?' So I took a big gulp and said, 'Okay, we'll do it.'

"That's how it started."

Where We Are Now

"Where we are now is not where we've been," concurs Steve Stites, MD, executive vice president of clinical affairs & chief medical officer at The University of Kansas Health System.

Since 2007, The University of Kansas Hospital has been ranked with the top hospitals in the country by *U.S. News & World Report*[19] Since 2010, when regional rankings were added to that report, KU Hospital has been the only one ranked number one in the Kansas City Metropolitan Area, and since 2012, when state rankings were added, the only one ranked number one in the State of Kansas.

With over 200 medical specialties available, approximately 290,000 unique patients[20] from every state in the country and many international locations were cared for at The University of Kansas Health System in fiscal year 2019. Nearly 2 million were seen for clinic and outpatient visits; 64,000 for hospital stays; 62,000 in the Emergency Department; and nearly 92,000 for surgical procedures at the vast main hospital campus in Kansas City, Kansas, and over 100 additional locations across the metropolitan area.

Statewide, Kansans have access to world-class care through all locations of The University of Kansas Health System. This includes locations in Overland Park, Topeka, Hays, Great Bend, and Larned.

Through the Care Collaborative that focuses on standardizing care and improving outcomes, The University of Kansas Health System partnership reaches further still with 72 hospitals, clinics, and EMS teams in 66 Kansas counties representing more than 60 percent of the state.

The story of The University of Kansas Health System's transformation provides more than a map. It's an atlas covering the vast areas that have to be navigated both functionally and philosophically to arrive at the epicenter—the heart—of the matter: the patient.

The University of Kansas Health System has been a consistently strong performer (4- or 5-star rating) for 14 out of 15 years of the Vizient/UHC Quality & Accountability Study.

Ranked as a 5-star performer out of 99 comprehensive academic medical centers in quality and patient safety for eight of fifteen years, and a 4-star performer for an additional six years,[21] The University of Kansas Health System has become a destination hospital for patients nationally and globally. We are...

- Consistently recognized in the *U.S. News & World Report* Best Hospitals rankings.
- The best hospital in the Kansas City Metro (11 years) and in Kansas (9 years)—the only hospital to have ever received these designations.
- In the top 1 percent of hospitals nationwide by being ranked in six or more specialties...[22]
    - Ear, Nose, and Throat
    - Geriatrics
    - Nephrology
    - Neurology and Neurosurgery
    - Pulmonology
    - Urology
- A *U.S. News* top 10 percent "high performer" in Cancer, Diabetes & Endocrinology, Orthopedics, Cardiology & Heart Surgery, and Gastroenterology & GI Surgery.[23]
- One of only 71 NCI-designated centers nationwide where patients have a 25 percent greater chance of survival.[24]
- One of only 3.9 percent of U.S. hospitals that have earned Magnet™ designation for nursing excellence three times in a row.
- The proud employer of the prestigious "Magnet Nurse of the Year" national award winners in 2012, 2014, and 2018.

- Ranked in the top 7 percent of hospitals nationwide recommended by patients surveyed by the Hospital Consumer Assessment of Healthcare Providers and Systems (HCAHPS).[25]
- The first heart care program in the nation to achieve The Joint Commission's Comprehensive Cardiac Center (CCC) Certification (in 2017).[26]
- A great place to work—turnover in nursing was 9.5 percent in 2019, which is over 40 percent lower than the national average.[27]
- The most highly ranked healthcare employer in Kansas by the *Forbes* America's Best Employers by State 2019 study.[28]

The chapters that follow detail the development of the leadership and business model that made this possible and sustainable—even during a pandemic. By applying lessons from world-class companies outside of healthcare, as well as the wisdom gained directly from lived-experience within this institution, The University of Kansas Hospital was transformed.

"Imagine" was the watchword Bob Page would use to draw a group into the vision that was—at one time—almost unimaginable. That vision—and its sustainability—became a reality.

LEADERSHIP LESSON:

Your job as a leader is to actualize the potential of your followers.

What it takes to turn an organization's death knell into an anthem is, in a word, leadership. And the leadership at the helm of KU Hospital's transformation had that synchronous combination of principles and skills. From Irene Thompson to Robert Hemenway and George Farha to Bob Page and Tammy Peterman to Scott Glasrud and Chris Hansen to Jon Jackson and more, theirs isn't a story of CEO-centrism or executive-directives, but "a story of the importance of leadership in actualizing the potential of its people," according to national healthcare consultant and Lean guru Mike Rona.[29]

"Repeatedly, from the beginning of their time, what was considered the impossible was made the target," Rona said of KU Hospital's transformation.

What was considered the impossible was made the target.

LEADERSHIP LESSON:

This is a story about the importance of key leadership values that seeded the culture for transformation with:

- Optimism and a belief in the "possible"
- Genuine commitment to whatever it takes to put the patient first
- Humility—not false humility, but a genuine belief that they could always be better
- Respect for those whom you serve and those with whom you serve
- Civility and compassion—you don't have to be a "jerk" to be an effective leader
- Administrative support and encouragement for innovation and inclusion
- Collaboration—where patient care is determined by an engaged and multidisciplinary team
- Belief in enabling the best in others while expecting the same of yourself
- Trust and confidence in leadership
- Joy in working together

How Better Becomes Best

After Irene Thompson moved on to become president and CEO of the University HealthSystem Consortium in 2007, the architecture of transition she had designed was expanded by a leadership team well positioned to take over. Thompson's choice to replace her as president and CEO was Bob Page. He asked Tammy Peterman, RN, to take on the roles of executive vice president, COO, and chief nursing officer (CNO).

Page's business savvy and Peterman's healthcare acumen were fused by strong mutual respect and trust in one another's competencies. As a team, they modeled the leap of faith necessary and deflected credit for the results their collaboration produced. Page and Peterman were admired inside the hospital and out in the community. A powerful but humble force, they didn't seek the institutional and personal accolades that mark their tenure. Rather, Page and Peterman were driven by a constancy of purpose: to be the best hospital in the nation and to reach that goal by putting patients and staff—not profits—first.

HOW WE KNOW THAT

Proud but Never Satisfied: The Leadership of Tammy Peterman

When I first came to this hospital, Tammy was the one who would take me up to the patient units and get me comfortable walking in and out of places. I remember the first time I walked into the Surgical Intensive Care Unit; I'd stick as close to the middle of the hallway as I could because those were really sick people in there with a lot of complicated equipment all around them. I wanted to connect with people, but I was scared to death. I had to get comfortable with patients.

I came to understand the value of talking to the patient and then going out and talking to the staff immediately. Then we would write notes to staff: *Thanks for the great work that you are doing.* There were some real simple things that we started to do but it was truly putting the right chief nurse in there that I think helped me get comfortable with patients and transformed nursing at this organization. That person was Tammy Peterman.

Some leaders are superficial. Tammy gets to know the people she works with—she truly connects with people. She is charismatic and inspirational. People listen to Tammy, believe in her, and want to follow her. She's also fun and knows how to have fun. Tammy is team-oriented and inclusive. She loves to surround herself with people—it has never been nor ever will be about herself.

She always does her best. One of her mantras is to *bloom where you are planted.* She is never satisfied. She is always looking for things she could do better. She is honest and has the highest level of integrity. She believes in others and always sees or looks for the best in other people. And she can let go of hard feelings quickly. Rarely does she write someone off completely—she doesn't hold grudges. Once she deals with a difficult situation, she is able to move on.

During my career, I have seen leaders who adopted certain characteristics to be successful (cut-throat, aggressive, etc.). Tammy has remained true to who she is as a person, and she's been extremely successful. She is incredibly humble, especially for a person who has achieved such national prominence. Tammy always wants to make sure she does the right thing. She has a well-defined moral compass and is always true to that compass.

Many people will tell you they learned what to do from their parents, and in this case, that's a very good thing. I believe the root of Tammy's principles and characteristics is her father who was a country doctor out in western Kansas. I had the privilege of meeting and getting to know him before he died. He was a kind, gentle, well-respected, and very successful man. In so many ways, Tammy is the next generation.
—Bob Page

HOW WE KNOW THAT

The Bold, Visionary Leadership of Bob Page

As I think about people who have supported and guided me in my executive career, Bob's part has been most significant. He is a great teacher—always explaining complex issues in terms easily understood. I have developed financial acumen over the years in executive roles, but initially needed someone to serve as my mentor—that person was Bob.

Bob is honest, ethical, and thoughtful. He's insightful and visionary—more than anyone I know. He's a big thinker—always aiming for the stars. We each have a "first, best, and only" list on our desk, and more than a few of those achievements started with Bob's vision and ideas. But he's also practical and consistent. Bob isn't afraid to put big, seemingly out of reach goals or ideas on the table. His vision of the Kansas Strategy for Healthcare was a bold concept. He truly believed we could re-engineer the healthcare delivery system statewide to improve the health of Kansans—and we're starting to do just that.

Being a huge sports fan, he created an annual "Hall of Fame"—a remarkable event where we celebrate those people and organizations that have been catalysts for our success. Another of those firsts was the creation of the Chiefs Fantasy Camp. Working with the president of the Kansas City Chiefs, Bob developed a one-and-only experience for Chiefs fans young and old to get a behind-the-scenes look at the action as well as participate as a player with coaching by Chiefs alumni. Funds generated from it support the KU Health System's Center for Concussion Management.

Not many people know Bob has taken a leadership role in promoting and sustaining the Negro Leagues Baseball Museum in Kansas City, serving as chair of fundraising and the committee to create awareness of the Hall of Fame induction events. He's generous with his time and always willing to help ideas with great potential take root. Bob even established an endowment fund for our rehabilitation department in honor of the care his mother received there. The Elizabeth Page Award for Excellence in Rehabilitative Care goes to one or two peer-nominated staff members annually and includes a monetary gift.

Bob treats everyone with the same degree of respect and courtesy. From the physicians to our staff, he's "Bob," never "Mr. Page." His code of behavior is innate and authentic—developed with a "service" mentality from his parents who were both in the military. He is a true servant leader.
—Tammy Peterman

LEADERSHIP LESSON:

What it takes to turn an organization's death knell into an anthem is, in a word, leadership.

When The University of Kansas Hospital committed to putting patients first in every decision back in 1998, it wasn't planting its flag on profitability as the priority—a risky position for a hospital that had just cut its source of sure income from the state. It was banking on the belief in a business model that hadn't been tested yet—to *Do the Right Thing*. Its success is a tribute to the leaders who imagined it, the guiding formula that made it work, and the culture that has sustained it.

The leadership of Page and Peterman brought all of that together, according to Susan Pingleton, MD. "It's like day and night," she said. "Before, there was never any focus. We weren't trying to make the patient unhappy, but there was not a focus at any level, among physicians, students, nurses, dietary—no one. That was just an inconceivable thought. So to have this as a priority, and then to educate, as we have heard virtually every employee has been educated, has made a difference."[30]

Pingleton said she saw it unfold as former chair of internal medicine at KUMC, but also on a personal level.

"A friend of mine was in the hospital for a knee replacement," she recalled. "I was with her most of the time. It is astonishing the culture of healthcare delivery in this hospital, with the number of people who touch the patient—even for a relatively simple procedure like that. She was in the hospital for four days, and I suspect 100 to 150 people touched her in some way, whether it was the person who brought meals, the person who took the blood pressure, or the students.

"Think of the magnitude—that you can inculcate every one of those people with a culture of 'How can I help; what can I do for you?' That's the culture right now," Pingleton concluded. "It's really quite dramatic."

CHAPTER TWO

Believe It

The only way to achieve the impossible is to believe it is possible.
—Alice Kingsleigh in *Alice Through the Looking Glass*

If Kayla Northrop, RN, believed in anything, it was in her own ingenuity. Lack of resources and repairs made workarounds the standard operating procedure at The University of Kansas Hospital in the '90s. She remembered, "The call lights were never functional on the burn unit where I worked," so she innovated.

Northrop set her chair in the middle of the open floor where she could keep an eye on patient beds along the walls while she was charting.

"No one had a room, just a curtain," she recalled. "I didn't want patients yelling out when they needed me because that would wake the person next to them, so I would leave a plastic cup on their bedside table with directions to knock it to the floor if the patient needed something. When I heard the noise, then I could see where it dropped and know where to go."

That was the nurse call button in the burn unit.

But the sea change at KU Hospital would make believers out of Northrop and over 2,000 other employees who decided not to abandon ship in 1998. CEO Irene Thompson and the senior leadership team were steadily turning the tanker with staff and patients on board. Once the Kansas Legislature approved Senate Bill 373 in 1998, The University of Kansas

Hospital set its own course. Everything that happened next would have to work, or they'd all be sunk.

While immediate operational issues had to be addressed just to keep the doors open, Thompson, Bob Page, Tammy Peterman, and the rest of the team knew the success of every endeavor depended on people, so priorities and processes were established with that in mind (See Chapter 3: Culture It and Chapter 5: Question It).

LEADERSHIP LESSON:

Success depends on people, so establish priorities and create processes accordingly.

From the trenches to the top levels of the organization, everyone had to understand and commit to the goal of being a hospital where people came first—starting with patients but including staff. To do that, they had to believe it was achievable. It was up to executive leadership to articulate the vision and galvanize an actionable plan to realize it.

Thompson's town hall meetings lit the "burning platform" while establishing a new commitment to transparent communication. The message generated the necessary tension for change, but once it had the desired effect, "Collectively, we had to shift to a positive outlook and lean into the possibilities," Bob Page stated.

LEADERSHIP LESSON:

Positivity is essential to inspire. Fear may compel action, but hope sustains it.

The problem was, no one knew what was possible. Lack of confidence among some key constituencies was understandable, given the long trend of decline.

"With every new CEO or chief nurse, we always had hope that we would have more staffing or that we would get better equipment," Nancy Martin, RN, recalled. "It was always a surprise when those things didn't happen." And now that the hospital no longer received funding from the state, all bets were off.

"I honestly didn't know if it would be possible, or even grasp how it was going to be possible," Kayla Northrop recalled. Her initial fears included, "Will I actually get a paycheck?"

I honestly didn't know if it would be possible...it felt like a momentous leap of faith, but hope changed the fear to trust.

Fortunately, Irene Thompson embodied a foundational tenet of leadership: She inspired confidence. Twenty years later, Thompson's words still came to mind for Clinical Quality Assurance Manager Paula Miller.

"She said, 'We can do this. You are great people,'" Miller remembered. "It was an exciting opportunity, and Irene presented it that way. She said, 'This is our last chance. We're going to hire the people we want at the right salary. And you're going to get the equipment you need when you need it—that's why we're doing this.'"

"We were all thinking, *She's serious!*" Miller added.

"It felt like a momentous leap of faith, but hope changed the fear to trust," said Northrop.

We're going to hire the people we want at the right salary. And you're going to get the equipment you need when you need it—that's why we're doing this.

Chris Ruder, RN, chief operating officer, Kansas City Division, had a similar recall. He was a unit manager at the time.

"I remember clearly the day I was called to meet with Irene, who was CEO then, along with several others including Bob Page and Scott Glasrud, who was the chief financial officer," said Ruder. "We were sitting there as she explained what it would take for each of us as leaders to help turn the hospital around. She told us we were not in a good place financially. Of course, we knew that."

Ruder steadied himself for the blow of bad news. But instead of the anticipated announcement of layoffs and Draconian cost-cutting measures, "Irene was clear that what would turn this around was to focus on making sure our nurses and the unit that we managed were providing the very best quality care and delivering the very best service to our patients and their families," Ruder recalled.

As simplistic as it was, the message was as unexpected as it was persuasive.

"I remember that day very distinctly—the conference room, the chair I was sitting in, and the discussion," Ruder said. "I think it truly was one of the cornerstone conversations that I had heard as a manager."

Former Chief Financial Officer Scott Glasrud concurred, "Our mantra from the beginning was, *You can't shrink your way to greatness.* We said the strategy is to grow, not slash and burn, and I think that resonated with people because morale was low. In terms of getting people on board, that was the most important message. We really believed it."

The strategy is to grow, not slash and burn, and I think that resonated with people because morale was low. In terms of getting people on board, that was the most important message. We really believed it.

Thompson and Page challenged every unit: *We believe in you; now show us what you can do.*

"It was not to go back and say, 'Irene said to do this,'" Ruder explained. "It was to help bridge communication so staff understood where we were and where our focus needed to be."

It was about engaging staff meaningfully in the dialogue about issues and solutions at relevant, actionable levels.

The effect was immediate. Across the hospital, what used to be an anxious buzz about more edicts coming down from on high was now the hum of everybody getting down to the business of planning how they'd meet this challenge in their department.

LEADERSHIP LESSON:

What would turn this around was to engage, charge, and trust the care team…to focus on making sure nurses had what they needed to provide the very best quality care to our patients and their families.

The Architecture of Transition

Cash

With only 30 days of cash, the question of where to start had no easy answer. Committees were established to work on governance, academic matters, financial relationships, property, administrative services, personnel, materials management, purchasing, media, and government relations.[1] Of paramount importance: getting cash into the coffers to fund everything.

"We had hardly any money to invest," Thompson explained. "The biggest change in cash came when we worked on our accounts receivable. We actually brought in some outside consultants to help us. We changed the whole system, and that brought a good deal of one-time cash to the bottom line, which gave us a bump."

Thompson took that edge to the rating agencies and was able to get a bond issue.

"I wasn't sure we would get rated because we were a new company," she recalled. "That's where my experience with Price Waterhouse and my familiarity with some of the raters really helped us. We were able to get a bond issue and begin to do some renovations and some badly needed work."

Malfunctioning lights in the operating rooms, the out-of-service foyer escalator, and leaky roofs were on the long list of problems that could now be addressed.

Capital Investment

"As we reinvested in facilities, we were viewed in the market as physician-friendly," Scott Glasrud said. "Word got out in the physician community that KU works with physicians, which wasn't necessarily the case with [competitors] Health Midwest or Saint Luke's."

Congenial relations with the physician community proved advantageous in many ways. Doctor referrals would build patient volume, which was crucial to every service line in the hospital. But two major issues had to be resolved before KUH could stabilize operations.

Distribution

First, the hospital's single urban location posed serious limitations for outpatient care. Irene Thompson and CIO Chris Hansen, who directed ambulatory services, solved that with the timely acquisition of a physician practice group with offices around the city.

"We had only one office off-site in 1998, and all other practices were sitting at our 39th and Rainbow Boulevard location," said Hansen. "So we bought TriSource Healthcare's medical group, and we named it Jayhawk Primary Care. Instantly, that took us from one practice of three docs to twelve locations with fifty-two docs off-site."

The new Jayhawk clinics increased patient access points.

"From a primary care perspective, Jayhawk Primary Care gave us the much larger footprint that we had to have," Tammy Peterman acknowledged.

Second, the crucial service lines of heart care and cancer treatment weren't viable in the existing KUH system, and the dynamics of both were complicated.

Service Lines

- **Cancer**

At the time of KU Hospital's spin-off in 1998, there were still 25 years remaining on the contract the university had signed with Salick Health Care, a California-based sub-contractor, to provide cancer treatment services.

"We couldn't make an investment in cancer because cancer is primarily an outpatient business, and (Salick) had our outpatient business," Thompson explained. "We shared the bottom line, but by the time all the overhead was allocated by Salick, there was no bottom line."

It was inconceivable for the hospital to move forward without a cancer program, so a long, difficult negotiation ensued. Eventually, an "out" was negotiated by KUH attorneys who informed Salick that the hospital wasn't legally obligated to maintain provider contracts with the university medical school. Lacking the hospital's clinical resources and setting, Salick couldn't operate, so a settlement was eventually reached.

Moving forward, the commitment to cancer treatment led KU Hospital to acquire the Kansas City Cancer Center directed by Dr. Mark Myron. After numerous conversations to explore the feasibility and fit between KCCC and KUH, Page, Peterman, and Myron were ready to proceed.

"I think the Kansas City Cancer Center acquisition worked because their leaders and their entire team focused a whole lot on the same things we do, which is making sure we're providing the very best care and support to patients. It's been highly successful," Peterman said.

KCCC brought more cancer patients and the ability to do more research because of the increased volume.

In 2011, the merged program provided the foundation to offer more patients clinical trials—an important component of The University of Kansas Cancer Center's earning NCI designation.

"I think that the merger with KU was a proud moment," Myron said. "We created a really great enterprise of cancer treatment for the whole community."

Today, Jeff Wright, vice president of cancer services, says, "The volume of blood-marrow transplant patients grew from 47 in 2007 to over 300, with patients now coming from across the U.S. and world for BMT and CAR T therapies."

- **Heart care**

"Kansas City needed a level-one trauma center," Thompson explained. "No one had it in the city, and a city this size should have that. We focused on that."

But it would be difficult to have an effective level-one trauma service without a heart program.

"We looked at many ways to try to solve that," said Thompson. "We had surgeons coming in from the community, but it was a catch-22 because cardiologists, to build their practice, needed to know that they had a strong surgical back-up. Surgeons want patients. You couldn't just put a lot of money into a surgeon and have him sit there all day until the cardiologists built up their practice."

Thompson's solution was an early indication of how KU Hospital would flex its new autonomy. She began meetings with Mid-America Cardiology (MAC) and Mid-America Thoracic and Cardiovascular Surgeons (MATCS), two large private practice groups that were severing their connections with KUH competitor St. Luke's. The resulting acquisition provided an immediate influx of physicians and patients that brought KU Hospital's plagued heart program back to life.

As with the Jayhawk acquisition, this entrepreneurial tact reflected Thompson's acute business sense that was already generating revenue in unprecedented ways. Although the transfusion of heart care professionals from private practice was met with some resistance by KU's School of Medicine, no one could argue with the immediate positive effects of the strategy.

Current KUMC Executive Vice Chancellor Rob Simari, MD, said, "It was an enlightened decision to bring MAC/MATCS on board; it was a turning point in the history of this hospital and health system. It was that decision upon which all ships rose."

The influence of MAC and MATCS immediately impacted patient care overall, because their practices had a very robust approach to customer service. They brought that with them, along with expectations of its implementation in the KUH setting.

"We gained a more organized system as a result of MAC-MATCS's coming and introducing theirs to us because they were so concerned about their patients having a good experience," said Thompson. "KU did not have an outstanding reputation in the community, and MAC-MATCS wanted to be sure that they could develop that here. They helped all of us grow and learn by putting new demands on us, which was good."[2]

What Business Are We In?

Although providing the very best quality care and delivering the very best service to patients and families was now the goal, the significance of it is best understood in contrast to its former tripartite agenda of research, education, and patient care. Since 1906, KU Hospital had been the clinical arm "providing a site for medical and biomedical research"[3] for the school of medicine at the University of Kansas Medical Center. Patient care was part of KUMC's mission, but given the university's focus on education and research, patients were often seen primarily for their income-generative potential, and therein lies the rub.

"When you are concentrating on clinical care, the patient ought to be your only interest," explained former COO Jon Jackson. "This campus had multiple experiences where that was not the case—where the care of the patient and the patient's interests were not first on the list, not second on the list, not third on the list, but were so far down the list as to be non-existent. That's why patient satisfaction was low."[4]

LEADERSHIP LESSON:

When you are concentrating on clinical care, the patient ought to be your only interest.

As an independent authority, KU Hospital could now prioritize its own list.

"We asked ourselves, *What business are we in?*" Bob Page recalled. In light of the hospital's poor performance—ranking in the 5th percentile for patient satisfaction nationwide in 1997—this wasn't a rhetorical question.

Tammy Peterman was hospital competency coordinator in 1998. She said, "The data showed we had poor patient satisfaction, so we felt this is where we should start. This is where we could make the biggest difference in the shortest amount of time."

But first, the issue of who would be treating those patients had to be ironed out. The physicians at KU Hospital were still contracted to KUMC, not to the hospital. And, as former KUMC health policy professor Arthur Daemmrich explained, "The hospital had to create its own identity without alienating the academic center. The key was to do this in a nuanced way so the physicians could retain their academic identity and link to the university while also doing patient care—the clinical enterprise."[5]

Identity work was certainly a priority, but the hierarchy of need was first to secure the official tie to the physicians so patients could be treated.

HOW WE KNOW THAT

The Most Important Thing We Do Is Save Lives

We had already determined our primary indicator for *service* was patient satisfaction, and the dial was moving in the right direction on that measure. But around 2001, I remember sitting down with the clinical department chairs during an off-site retreat discussing how we would define *quality* in this organization. We tossed many different ideas around before concluding that *all* quality indicators are important—reduction in falls, short wait time in the Emergency Department, swift transfer to the cath lab for cardiovascular patients, and a thousand other things.

Ultimately, we decided the most important indicator of quality in our hospital is the number of lives we save. The hospital leaders and the medical staff leaders agreed that was what we would call our "big dot" in quality. At the time this work began, we didn't have an accurate method for calculating lives saved. What we knew was our gross mortality ranged from 2.5 percent to 3.0 percent and was higher than the state and local averages.

In 2003, using data obtained from University HealthSystem Consortium (UHC), we were finally able to get a clear picture of our opportunity to "save lives" using the mortality index, a measure of hospital performance recognized industry-wide. Basically, the mortality index is a ratio of the actual number of hospital deaths during a specific period divided by the predicted number of deaths. This takes into account the patients' level of illness and outcomes for similar patients at hospitals across the country. We knew we'd have really strong metrics in all the areas we care so much about if our mortality index was low.

In 2004, KUH's mortality index showed 42 more deaths than would be normal or expected at our hospital. As an academic medical center that sees the sickest of sick patients, the challenge was huge. Even when adjusted (i.e., the "risk-adjusted mortality rate" or RAMR) for factors like the severity of the illness, our RAMR just reinforced how much improvement was needed.

You can't fix that unless everybody in your organization is working toward the same goal. And for us, patient outcomes are everyone's responsibility.

Some of us have nothing to do with providing direct care to a patient clinically. But I will tell you the one thing that remains critical to our quality outcomes has been this focus. Because of the strength of our rapid response teams and other innovations we've implemented, our quality metrics have improved. The partnerships between the medical leaders, the nursing leaders, and the intensive care units have all helped reduce deaths in our hospital.

Today, we have an organization in which even the staff in finance are held to the same bar as our clinical staff. They receive the same customer service training and function according to the culture code we've established. In fact, everyone in an executive or leadership role system-wide is evaluated with the same patient satisfaction goals. You might ask, "Why do you do that?" It's because those people in finance also walk the halls. If they see somebody who's lost, they can get that patient from point A to point B or help a family member. They're answering the phone when someone is trying to figure out how to pay their bill. There are many ways to impact the quality of the patient experience.

Between November 2005 and May 2020 at our health system, 3,436 patients lived who, statistically speaking, would have died based on their diagnosis and underlying conditions. We're living proof the bar can be set high, and it can be achieved.
—Tammy Peterman

The Doctor May Or May Not Be In

At the time of the Authority in 1998, the affiliation agreement between KUMC and KUH did not address the role and relationship of the physicians to the hospital.[6] The physicians were organized under Kansas University Physicians, Inc. (KUPI). KUPI was contracted by KUMC to provide for all the necessary business and back-office aspects of physician services. Historically, KUPI worked out the logistics of those arrangements with 18 specialized medical departments at The University of Kansas Hospital.

So physicians were employed not by the hospital per se, but by foundations (tax-exempt 501(c)(3) organizations) associated with their respective clinical department. In essence, surgeons worked for the department of surgery's foundation; the orthopedists were employed by the orthopedics foundation, and so on and so forth.

From department to department, a myriad of KUPI-managed contracts for physician services directed each "practice plan" (how physicians within a department or group share income) without consistency of process or equity in compensation. Now that the Authority was in place, KUPI had to re-contract these services with KU Hospital. It wasn't going to be easy.

"There was no uniformity to those deals," Bob Page noted. "You can imagine if you're Tammy or me or Scott Glasrud, there's a knocking at the door and you've got all these people wanting to negotiate the best deal possible."

Streamlining that process would take years to accomplish, but by 2006, negotiations were completed and contracts in place.

LEADERSHIP LESSON:

There has to be consistency and equity in the process for hiring, compensating, contracting, servicing, supplying, and administering the system-wide functions of a hospital.

Meanwhile, the patient care priority got a boost from what former CFO Scott Glasrud called "a fortuitous market phenomenon." Glasrud even "wondered whether we could have pulled it off without this phenomenon. It was the fact that there was this backlash to narrow networks."

Essentially, insurance companies pushing customers into a "narrow network" of HMOs (health maintenance organizations) limited their healthcare options. The eventual public pushback forced "the market to become a consumer-driven, open-access market, more PPO-driven [preferred provider organization] rather than HMO-driven," explained Glasrud. "Because of that, many of the changes we made could take effect, and we could reap the benefit of it," Glasrud continued. "People were freer to vote with their feet and come to a place that was focusing on the patient."[7]

Seeing Is Believing

Making good on each deliverable—updated equipment, the Jayhawk expansion, the heart care program, facilities repair, the cancer center, and equitable physician contracts—strengthened trust in leadership and the credibility of KU Hospital's new identity.

Each initiative provided tangible evidence of the administration's commitment to the vision first articulated in the town hall meetings. As the hospital became more functional, the form it was taking necessarily followed. In a dynamic that typified the process of infrastructural development at KU Hospital, form always followed function. Each endeavor was vetted in practice—weeding out what didn't work—before it was implemented system-wide.

"Particularly in the early days, we didn't always have time to get everything perfect before moving," Page said. "Sometimes it was 'ready, fire, aim' as we trialed what would work. There are always 180 degrees of potential right and 180 degrees of potential wrong. We weren't afraid to get it wrong, because that just eliminated an approach that wasn't right."

Getting it wrong was important to the process of learning what was right.

"One of our first attempts missed the mark," Page recalled. "Our initiative to improve patient satisfaction began by targeting the survey questions most highly correlated to overall satisfaction." Channeling David Letterman's *Top 10*, Page remembered telling leadership, "'All we need to do is focus on being more sensitive to how it feels to be in the hospital; being more concerned about privacy and being cheerful would move the dial.' While it got the conversation going, it didn't help our teams understand how to exemplify those behaviors, and ownership wasn't really established. And, it didn't really change the patient experience."

The chapters that follow elucidate what did work.

LEADERSHIP LESSON:
Form always follows function in a dynamic where each endeavor is vetted in practice before it's systematized.

Anything that didn't uphold the vision would be rejected. The University of Kansas Hospital would provide the best patient experience and outcomes—even if it was going to take some time and effort to figure out how to do that.

Sometimes it was "ready, fire, aim" as we trialed what would work. There are 180 degrees of potential right and 180 degrees of potential wrong. We weren't afraid to get it wrong, because that just eliminated an approach that wasn't right.

From the university side, head and neck surgeon Doug Girod, who would become chancellor of the University of Kansas in 2017, watched in admiration as it evolved.

"If you look at only revenues and efficiencies, you start viewing every person as a liability as opposed to an asset," he said.[8]

Instead of profit margins, the goal of all hospital operations was to create a better patient experience, both in terms of outcomes and satisfaction. Quality should be measured in that context.

"Theirs was just a really different approach to a business model," Girod said.

LEADERSHIP LESSON:
If you look at only revenues and efficiencies, you start viewing every person—whether patient or employee—as a liability as opposed to an asset. Instead of profit margins, our goal was to create a better patient experience, both in terms of outcomes

and satisfaction. Quality should be measured in that context. Our philosophy was if we've got that right, the rest will follow.

The question was how to get quality right based on evidence. Creating and sustaining the patient-centric culture while producing viable performance measures pushed the leadership team into new territory. Applying quality standards would have been an obvious method, but "at the time, the industry didn't have quantifiable measures of quality," Bob Page said.

The risk-adjusted mortality rate (RAMR) was considered the comparable indicator of how a hospital was performing. In 1998, the RAMR at KU Hospital was 1.14—14 percent higher than expected. Read: More deaths occurred at KUH than would be typical for an institution with this acuity. There was a lot of work to be done.

Thompson, Page, and Peterman sat down with all the clinical chairs and started the conversation: *Let's talk about quality. How will we know our care is evidence-based and achieving the highest levels of quality?*

As Tammy Peterman saw it, "Focusing on the quality of patient care would make us better clinicians. Quality outcomes would improve once we started measuring it, because we would know right away what was or wasn't working based on actionable performance."

It was a seminal point that intensified the need for data. And data is what the hospital didn't have, at least not any that could move the needle indicating improvement.

Theirs was just a really different approach to a business model.

Historically, KU Hospital mailed surveys to patients after discharge. Those that were completed and mailed back were bundled-off for processing to Press Ganey, an independent survey vendor. Press Ganey then generated quarterly reports, but the results were based on the date the survey had been returned, not on the date the care was provided.

"By the time we got it and could analyze it, the data was at least three to four months old—it was essentially useless," Page noted.

That wasn't going to work. It didn't support the vision, so Page brought the process in-house.

LEADERSHIP LESSON:

The goal of all hospital operations was to create a better patient experience, both in terms of outcomes and satisfaction. Quality should be measured in that context, and the performance data has to be shared widely.

The new process was begun in 2002, according to Chief Culture Officer Terry Rusconi, and involved "entering the survey data based on date of care into our own spreadsheet before sending the surveys onto Press Ganey to determine our benchmark performance."

The scores provided much-needed time-sensitive information.

"One of the concepts was that we are going to measure it, and we are going to report it, and we will see whether the numbers are good or bad," Page explained. "If it's bad, we are going to fix it. And if it's good, we are going to reward it. We were not an organization that was used to rewarding things and celebrating things."

That, too, was changing.

Looking Up

There were already indications that KUH was moving in the right direction. The University HealthSystem Consortium (now Vizient) collected data—by physician and patient—from most academic medical centers nationwide that KU Hospital could use to compare itself to other AMCs.

"We would identify where our trouble spots and outliers were," Irene Thompson said. KU Hospital was getting up to speed in key areas.

Moving in the Right Direction: Patient Satisfaction[9]

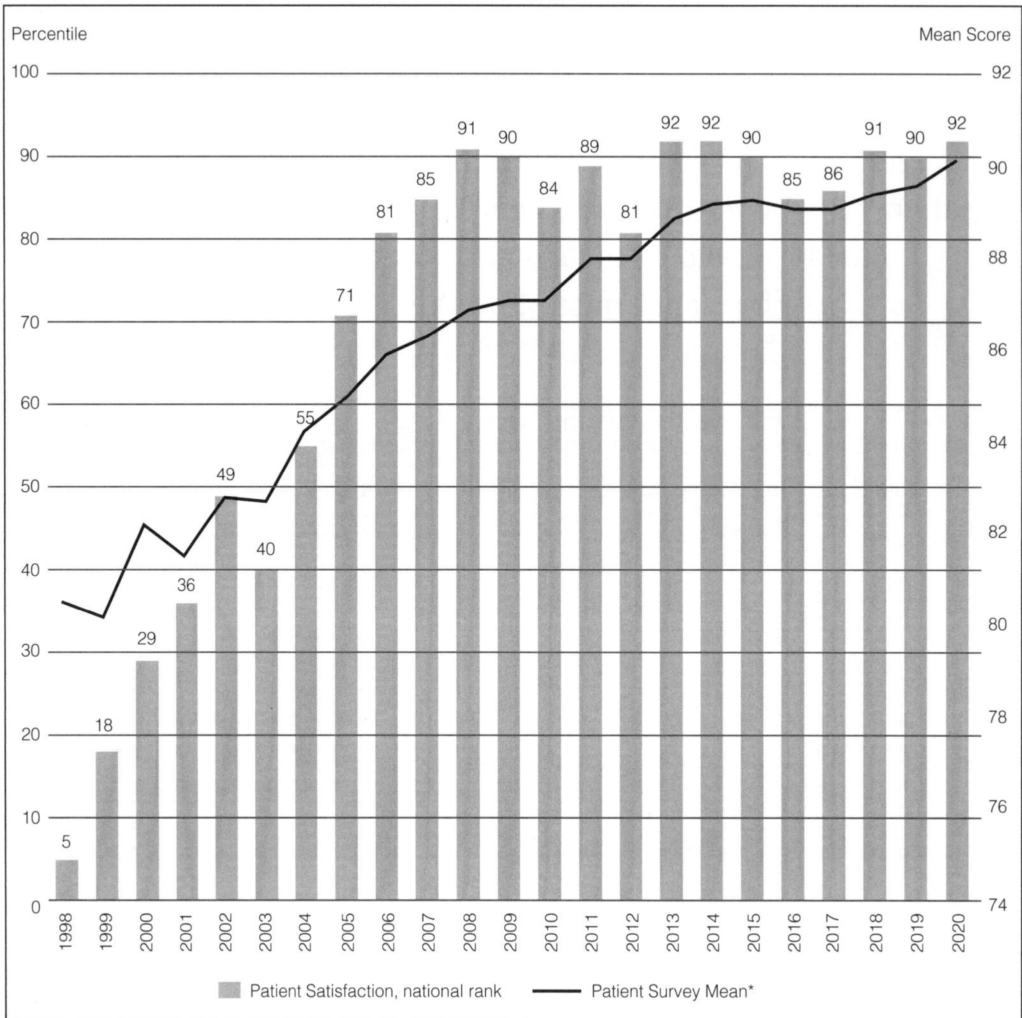

*Mean for calendar year out of maximum score of 100.

HOW WE KNOW THAT

Getting the Formula Right

As we started gaining momentum, other academic medical centers started asking, "What are you guys doing?" That forced us to stop and reflect.

In 2001, we were fortunate to work directly with Quint Studer and apply the lessons he had learned in transforming the cultures of two healthcare organizations to enhance our cultural and organizational improvement work.

In formulating our answer, we realized we'd fully embraced the five pillars Quint introduced to us and adapted them to our own culture. The pillars became stars to reinforce the responsibility of each member of the team for five-star performance. Navigating by those stars, a business model emerged, showing a cause-and-effect relationship between three principles foundational to our organization—service, quality, and people—and the growth and financial outcomes we needed to achieve.

On paper, the essence of the equation is quite simple:

Quality + Service + People = Growth + Sustainability

The core idea being, if we provide every patient with the best quality and service possible and we maintain the right team of people capable of delivering that level of care, everything else will take care of itself in terms of profitability. We don't fixate on growth or cost, but focus on the patient instead.

The Five-Star Guiding Formula

World-Class Patient Outcomes (Quality)
+
World-Class Patient Satisfaction (Service)
Delivered by Competent, Committed, and Engaged Staff (People)
=
Strong, Sustainable Growth (Strategic Growth)
+
Sustainable Financial Performance (Financial Sustainability)

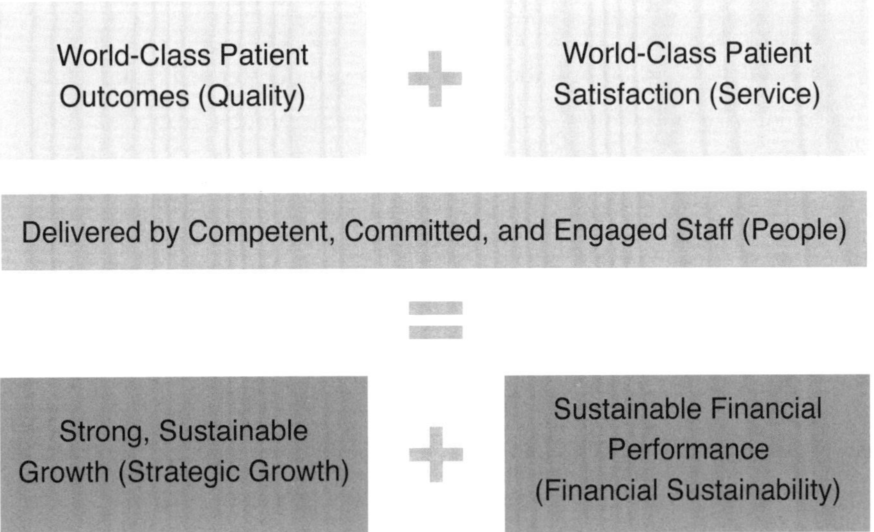

> The philosophy was if we've got that right, the rest will follow. Staying grounded in this vision—not on profit goals—means our formula never has to change, even when the market varies or the numbers change; it's still relevant and accurate. When we go back and look at the transformation of this organization, we can prove it time and time again. This is the formula that did it, and that's what we still live by.
> —Bob Page

Mission in a Model

If we have a business model, it's *Do the Right Thing*.

The Five-Star Guiding Formula directed KUH's emerging business model—at least to the extent there was one. Traditional profit-driven approaches to running a business didn't drive the process—functions vetted by the vision and goal did.

"If we have a business model, it's *Do the Right Thing*," acknowledged Bob Page. "And that was expressed in our Five-Star Guiding Formula."

Profit margins were a consideration, but only in context to patient-driven care.

"When money is the most important goal, things get sidestepped," said Doug Gaston, CFO and senior vice president since 2017. "Safety and process might be compromised. If you're all about making more money, you'll start lowering the standards on expensive investments like training, equipment, and human resources so you can save money in those areas. That's not in the best interests of patients."[10]

LEADERSHIP LESSON:

If every patient has the best experience and outcome possible, and if we maintain the right team of people capable of delivering that quality of care, everything else will take care of itself—including profitability.

Former CFO Scott Glasrud described the guiding formula as a "balanced scorecard" of progress toward goals in all five fronts of the organization.

"It's an overall philosophy of operating a major academic medical center," Glasrud explained. "We were trying to be a high performer in each area. The financial 'star' was not an end goal in itself, but rather a support to allow achievement of all the other stars."

As a business model, *Do the Right Thing* would be put to the test again and again as the hospital reinvented itself.

Put It to the Test

Early on, the organization had to choose the electronic medical record system that would be adopted across the clinical practice. Physicians, nurses, and other staff were invited to vendor demonstrations and asked to rank them. A number of factors, including ease of use, patient safety, and accessibility of information, were considered. Among the strong contenders were a local company and a more affordable option.

After due deliberation, the recommendation by all user groups was neither of those, but the one they felt would best support safe, effective, and patient-centered care. It was the right choice...and the system selected is still in place today.

Doing the right thing was demonstrated again with the health system's commitment to ensuring access to behavioral health. Anyone involved in healthcare knows reimbursement for behavioral healthcare is not optimal, and many organizations have opted to close their behavioral health facilities.

Understanding the community impact of those reductions in behavioral health resources, KU Health System stepped forward. In 2015, the organization took over operations of a pediatric acute psychiatric hospital and began expanding services at that location. TUKHS made a similar commitment to adult behavioral health, investing millions of dollars to create a state-of-the-art facility that opened its doors in 2019 on the health system's new Strawberry Hill campus in downtown Kansas City, Kansas.

Too often, an organization's vision remains theoretical or esoteric. But the Five-Star Guiding Formula actually operationalized KU Hospital's vision. As a synergic equation, it both inspired and prescribed the functional evaluation for each of the five performance categories.

This model guided the organization's vision and mission as it evolved from hospital to health system.

> This health system has a clear focus on its purpose: high-quality care of the patient. We invest in outstanding care, and that requires advanced technology and involvement in clinical trials that lead to new treatments such as those we're doing with CAR-T. What we have always said is technology is only as good as what it does to help improve patient care and outcomes. We won't and don't chase technology for technology's sake like some organizations do.
>
> By having a clear, singular focus on patient care, the financial end takes care of itself. Obviously, we need financial solvency, but that's not what drives operations here. Our financial goals are designed to give us the sustainability to achieve our broader goals of providing the best care and outcomes for patients. The financial piece of the equation is important, but it's not the most important thing. Finance alone doesn't dictate our goals. Our financial goals are designed to support our mission.
> —Doug Gaston, CFO and Senior Vice President

Believing Your Vision Statement

Since it was initially established as the laboratory where the University of Kansas students learned their medical trade in 1905, the hospital's vision and mission were fixed to that purpose when it opened in 1906. Its identity was understood as support to education and research functions until KUH gained independence from the state in 1998.

While the mission began to reflect patient-centered values in '98, it was still heavily focused on the education of health professionals. That didn't change much in a 2002 rewrite, although greater emphasis was given to enhancing health and wellness; the vision remained a lackluster *To be the center for advanced medicine.*

Things began to change in 2008 when the hospital formally committed to a vision of becoming a national leader in caring, healing, teaching, and learning. Fully embracing clinical integration in 2016, and its new name by 2017, The University of Kansas Health System modified *learning* to *discovering* in its updated statement.

To be a national leader in caring, healing, teaching, and discovering articulated KU Health System's cultural foundations for staff, physicians, the community, the region, and the state.

LEADERSHIP LESSON:
To lead the nation requires leadership that has earned its followership.

Easier Done Than Said

If an organization's identity is represented in its name, The University of Kansas Hospital had an identity crisis.

"We've had multiple names over the number of years since the beginning of the Authority," said Terry Rusconi, who has had numerous titles himself during his tenure at KU Health System—from VP of performance improvement to chief culture officer. "For most of the early years, you'd hear 'The University of Kansas Hospital' or 'KU Med.' That was primarily because the community knew us—and still refers to us—as KU Med."

With the acquisition of the Jayhawk Group, and eventually other acquisitions and affiliations with hospitals across Kansas, "The University of Kansas Hospital," or the "Authority," or "The University of Kansas Hospital Authority," or "KU Hospital," as it has variously been called, was far more than a physical structure on the KUMC campus at 39th and Rainbow Boulevard in Kansas City, Kansas. To reflect that growth, the name began transitioning in 2012 to "The University of Kansas Health System," which was formally adopted by 2017.

Until that finally happened, "it was pretty confusing internally and externally," Rusconi admitted. "That's how it started."

All of this would find its best and highest expression in the unique culture of this organization.

CHAPTER THREE

Culture It

Culture is not an initiative. Culture is the enabler of all initiatives.
—Larry Senn

No one had seen anything like it since the influenza pandemic of 1918. Ashleigh Adams, RN, admitted she was scared. On the front lines at KU Health System in the spring of 2020, she was bearing up with the other nurses, but the situation was far from easy.

"We had conversations," Adams said. "*Are you scared?* Because I'm scared."

"Normally, I've got this—like the back of my hand," she added. "But with COVID-19, it was changing every hour. Sometimes you had to step away from the bedside and have a breathing moment."

Adams worked directly with COVID-19 patients and experienced the strain like everyone else, but also felt bolstered by the support that typifies the culture of this health system. Even before COVID-19 cases were identified in the Kansas City area, KU Health System was reaching out to organizations where the pandemic had hit to understand what kind of support their staff needed. As the health system braced itself with a surge plan for incoming patients, it simultaneously created an infrastructure to address emotional, psychological, and practical needs and to provide resources to support resilience for staff and providers.

The resiliency and support team offered up a wide array of tools and events to help employees cope.

"Change is destabilizing, and during this crisis, every day was characterized by change," said Gregory Nawalanic, PsyD, clinical psychologist at TUKHS. "Organizational agility is important, both functionally and psychologically. Our psychologists and chaplains introduced a series of supportive calls where folks could share, in a safe space, the things they are going through. We accommodate up to ten front-line staffers at a time, to support them and give them a chance to express their feelings and anxieties."[1]

These sessions were scheduled every day at the times most convenient for staff working days or nights, and staff members used a code to call into the conversation.

"It was a chance to discuss things we needed and just speak to how we were doing overall," Adams said. The sessions were incredibly helpful for her.

The team also researched, curated, and published a dedicated web-link on the site's landing page that connected to articles, resilience tools, and targeted resources for staff. They created plans to help staff address basic needs at home, such as potential housing, grab-n-go foods or home food and grocery delivery, and dry-cleaning support. They also expanded the call-in sessions to reach larger, team-based groups wanting to process feelings and experiences with peers. For Adams, that was huge.

"It's nice to be able to talk to someone and say, 'This is how I'm feeling'...it's nice!" she said.

Cultural Resilience

Response to a crisis of epic proportion is arguably the greatest test of any organizational culture.

"Our crisis and care practices draw from direct experience with Ebola, H1N1, and other highly communicable novel diseases, so we have a plan," Tammy Peterman said.[2]

Still, because each health threat is unique, the health system's ready plan came with willingness to change it as needed.

Adapting to particular, even rare, circumstances requires agility and resiliency. Both are manifested in the organization's culture.

"You can't invent a resilient organization in response to the urgent need for one," Bob Page affirms. "If you've got the culture right, it will support you in a crisis. In fact, it'll save lives."

Belief + Behavior = Culture

When every mind melds on the same goal—like the commitment made back in 1998 to put patient needs first—group action in a crisis can be swift and agile. Each individual is bringing his or her expertise and a sense of personal ownership to the challenge.

Tammy Peterman expressed it this way: "Thinking as an individual while acting as a team is our culture in action."

Thinking as an individual while acting as a team is our culture in action.

Being of service is the nature of the people who work here. The combination of belief and behavior permeates the culture of The University of Kansas Health System. If you ask a staff member or a physician for an example of this culture in action, you'll get a ready, very real response.

"I remember one patient who came to us not knowing he had liver disease—just that he got really sick, really fast," recalled Sean Kumer, physician vice president for perioperative and procedural services and surgical director for liver transplantation. "And he had no insurance, which was another level of complication. He came into the Intensive Care Unit, and we got him on lifesaving support with an artificial liver-assist device.

"While the ICU docs and nurses were taking care of this patient, the transplant surgeons were working with the ICU team to get him listed for a transplant," added Kumer. "And the financial folks were working hard on getting him some insurance. In the end, we saved his life. It was a huge team effort from a ton of people. A week after his transplant, this young gentleman walked out of this hospital into a whole new life. It was so gratifying."

It's a culture that hinges on trust and partnership—each member of the team owning his or her part—plus a little bit more so nothing gets missed. It's a culture that imbues bedside staff with the authority to do the right thing for each patient. It's about empowering frontline leadership and representative leadership at administrative levels. The egalitarian consistency is a hallmark of this culture.

"It's all oars pulling in the same direction," said Terry Rusconi. "The synergy strengthens the effort, so better outcomes are achieved faster, and patients have a better experience."

"The most important factor in the transformation of this hospital has been our culture," CEO Bob Page observed. "Employees aren't loyal to strategy; they're loyal to a culture they've contributed to and are a part of. If they believe in its vision and values, your people are your strongest advocates. In my opinion, we're positioned better than most because we got our culture right."[3]

LEADERSHIP LESSON:

Employees aren't loyal to strategy; they're loyal to a culture they've contributed to and are a part of. If they believe in its values, your people become your strongest advocates.

For The University of Kansas Hospital, that vision was to create an institution where patients had the best experience and outcomes--better than at any other healthcare institution in America. It would require providing quality and service at a level KUH had never before achieved—performing with the best of the best in the nation. It wouldn't happen overnight, but the cultural shift toward that goal began as soon as the institution became independent in 1998.

"We were committed to being the kind of hospital that put people first—starting with our patients and including our staff as well," Tammy Peterman explained. "That meant being laser-focused on quality at every level—building and supporting a competent and committed team. To deliver the best patient experience and outcomes, we had to start by having the right people on board. That was one of the 'five stars' in our guiding formula."

The X-Factor in Culture

After separating from the state system, staff who remained at KUH was understandably anxious. Leaping from the known world into the unknown creates apprehension—even if what's ahead looks promising. Employees had been familiar with the hospital's dysfunction, but were unsure of their ability to meet new expectations. Bolstering confidence was a complicated process.

"We had to build safety nets between the old and new cultures," Bob Page explained.

LEADERSHIP LESSON:

We had to build safety nets between the old and new cultures.

This would take form through a myriad of functional innovations. Identifying a 20-year veteran of the hospital's clinical laboratory as the face of customer service was one of them.

As a newly independent organization, every employee at KU Hospital had to be on-boarded system-wide in 1998. Whether a long-time department director or a just-hired custodian, a new grounding in patient-centered care had to be assimilated by all staff. It was a massive undertaking, but instead of outsourcing the training, Bob Page took a novel approach. He decided to capitalize on something that was already working really well: the exceptional patient focus and congeniality of Paula Miller, a clinical laboratories department leader.

"Paula had a very important job in our lab, and we noticed that everyone enjoyed working with her," Page explained. "Every day, she modeled the kind of customer service orientation that we wanted from all our employees."

The thinking was, "If everyone treated people the way Paula did, we'd have a customer service-oriented operation," Tammy Peterman said.[4]

Asking a laboratorian to take over customer service training was a defining moment for the organizational culture.

"It's not just what she's saying when she orients new employees; it's who she is that adds meaning to the message," Page explained. "It shuts down the 'things like that don't happen' presumption of this industry. We had to have the right person in that job who understood the culture of this hospital."

Miller took a week to consider the offer, then signed on enthusiastically. Page encouraged her to infuse the training with her passion. The curriculum needed full immersion in the emerging KUH culture.

We had to have the right person in that job who understood the culture of this hospital. It's not just what she's saying when she orients new employees; it's who she is that adds meaning to the message.

Customer service training began in 1999. True to what would become the norm for the system, this mission-critical initiative started at the top level of the organization. Executive leaders and senior managers were the first to go through not only the eight-hour customer service course all staff would receive, but also eight hours of instruction on how to lead in a service environment prior to rollout of training to others in the organization. "This would ensure their ability to support and reinforce the expectations being established through the training process," Tammy Peterman said.

Hiring Culture

Today, that training curriculum has expanded, and so has the hiring process that's calibrated to find "the X-factor" in candidates who are a good fit for this culture. That process includes:

- Training managers on behavior-based interviewing (BBI) strategies
- Incorporating peer interview experiences

- Enhancing the role of the talent acquisition team to ensure fit and alignment with the culture
- Filtering not just for skill but for will

Once hired, the on-boarding process was enhanced so orientation and integration into the work group and organization engaged the hearts, souls, and minds of new teammates. What used to be a singular event expanded longitudinally from the interview process, through offer, through the time between offer and start date, then with orientation and introduction to the new work area.

At every new employee orientation, Bob Page and Tammy Peterman address new employees. Their message is a mix of inspiration, challenge, and validation. When Page says, "You have been carefully selected to be a part of this," he's not being effusive. The KU Health System hiring process is exacting.

"We hire the best person—and that begins with making sure he or she understands and can embrace our culture," said Tammy Peterman. "We can help develop technical competency, but that X-factor is the ability to be successful in this culture. That's what we're looking for in every candidate."

Today, this customized training is still required for all new employees. It spans a full day covering the culture code of The University of Kansas Health System. Over the years, proposals to shorten the training have been nixed. Eight hours of instruction focused on the culture of service that all employees have to attend sends a very clear message about what's important.

"If you're here just for yourself or the Friday paycheck, this might not be the place for you," Paula Miller said. "We had one new employee who fell asleep during orientation—that was his first and last day on the job. People figure it out really quick."

Those who fully engage often describe a sense of calling to this work. They want to work for a hospital that matches their passion for helping patients. And Miller was quick to add, "Guess what—your coworker likes to be treated with kindness and respect, just like patients do. Your coworker is your customer, too."[5]

LEADERSHIP LESSON:

Guess what—your coworker likes to be treated with kindness and respect, just like patients do. Your coworker is your customer, too.

Kayla Northrop, burn program coordinator, has been employed at KU Hospital since 1990. She remembers going through Miller's training.

"Some of us call it 'Happy Class'—but endearingly," Northrop laughed. "Kindness and caring are an expectation within our culture. We're going to hold the elevator door or take time to make a connection—it is just what we do."

Cultivating a Culture

Getting and keeping the right people on the bus was vital, so the job application and review processes were calibrated accordingly. The best and brightest were always sought, but the most important factor was and continues to be the cultural fit. *Why did this candidate want to be here? What has he or she done in past roles and positions that indicates a passion for taking great care of customers and being a great teammate? How does the team feel this individual would fit into and support the department's critical work?* All of these factors were part of the behavior-based interviewing process developed and implemented in the early years of the Authority.

"Our people built this culture," Peterman said. "As leaders, our job is to ensure this culture is sustained so our staff can invest their time, talent, and passion into what it takes to achieve world-class patient care."

Everything revolves around the goal of putting the patient first so, "We want our employees to find new and better ways of doing things," Bob Page explained. "We actively encourage curiosity and breakthrough thinking. And it's up to leadership to cultivate and maintain an environment that supports that."

LEADERSHIP LESSON:

When everything revolves around putting the patient first, it's essential that staff can trust leadership to provide what's needed to achieve that goal.

The strategies for doing that were vetted by the culture itself.

Culture with Strategy

The University of Kansas Hospital leveraged every opportunity to define and reinforce its culture. Strategies to bring leadership and followership into closer, more effective communication and connection strengthened it in a variety of ways.

"Here at KU Health System, when we round, we round as a team," explained Joseph McGuirk, MD. "That approach has been cultivated here. The physician, the nurse practitioner, the pharmacist, and the nurse who's taking care of that patient—I won't round without the nurse. If the nurse is busy, we'll hold off and come back. We'll go find that nurse if s/he's not on the floor. Then together, we go through the problem list—what is our plan for the day? Everybody has input. That's just a no-brainer—it's what you'd expect a healthcare team to be doing."[6]

- **Management Rounding**

  Management rounding ensured access to leadership from staff on the front lines—even on the late shift. Marilyn Rymer, vice president of neurosciences at KU Health System, was among those from the organization's leadership team who did nighttime rounds with staff working in clinical and non-clinical settings.

  "The leadership would come in after 9:00 p.m.," she said. "We were assigned a place to go in the hospital. We'd usually go in pairs and have a set of questions that we asked. One night, I was on one of the units and we were supposed to ask if the staff had everything they needed so they were able to do their work. We heard a lot! 'Yes, during the day things are fine. But on nights and weekends, you could make some improvements.'

"So we took back all their suggestions and operationalized those that we could," Rymer recalled. "I never saw anything like that happen anywhere else I've worked. I never saw any interest from the senior leadership team in asking the physicians or staff on a ward about what could be better."

McGuirk concurs. "This is the exception, not the rule, in our nation. We have major healthcare-associated problems and infections in patients nationwide because team medicine is not being done."[7]

- **The Solutions Room**

  An innovation called the "Solutions Room" was a real-time, 24-hour help line established in 2003 to systematize policies and processes. The phone line was answered around the clock, seven days a week, by trained representatives—all members of the hospital's management team. The goal was to have a go-to source for help if a first call to a department or individual did not generate the needed results. Indeed, the most common (67.1 percent) issues were the inability of systems and processes (across many areas) to meet the needs of staff providing patient care. Staff education and training needs comprised 17.4 percent of the calls, and 15.5 percent were isolated/one-time issues linked to a special cause, such as a patient needing a battery for his hearing aid.

The Solutions Room was especially busy on nights and weekends when there wasn't a manager on the unit or senior leadership in the supporting departments. Situations ranging from missing telephones to patient bed placement to unique requests made by individual patients were all problem-solved in the Solutions Room.

"When an issue was successfully resolved, the representative would call the customer back to confirm satisfaction and close the loop," explained Terry Rusconi.

The Solutions Room not only provided timely support to staff, it helped executive leadership understand the challenges on the front line where support mechanisms weren't agile or substantial enough to meet the growing needs of the hospital.

"If the same problem emerged in three different places, we knew it wasn't situational; we had to address the issue systemically," Page explained.

This program continued until functional systems were in place to support staff.

- **Inpatient Operating System**
  Improving the experience of patients and staff at KU Health System meant redefining the improvement process itself. The resulting Inpatient Operating System (IOS, see Chapter 6) is a groundbreaking innovation that changed the role of management, developed self-directional teams on each unit, and raised the bar on outcomes for patient safety and satisfaction. The IOS model has proven sustainability, and is being implemented hospital-wide.

  "The IOS happened because we have a continuously improving culture that looks proactively for opportunities to do better," said Chris Ruder, RN, chief operating officer, Kansas City Division.

- **Affirmation and Celebration**
  The importance of affirming and celebrating what's going right can't be overstated. It can't be limited to epic events, and it must be pervasive throughout the culture. Celebration as a strategy is a very big deal at KU Health System since its humble beginnings with a candy cart during third-shift rounds by the executive team. Celebration culture grew out of a desire to make The University of Kansas Hospital a better place to work. (See Chapter 9 for the leadership lessons that *Celebrate It.*)

"Culture outperforms strategy every time, and culture with strategy is unbeatable." —Quint Studer

HOW WE KNOW THAT

Operationalizing Our Culture

One of the most important things we did post-Authority to embed our cultural values into our operation was change how we documented and communicated about patient care. We had a mostly paper-based process that was antiquated and unsafe—there were lots of black holes; necessary information might not reach its intended recipient. We'd been told by our Joint Commission survey consultant that our clinical documentation system wasn't safe and wouldn't meet The Joint Commission (TJC) standards. We needed a cutting-edge, safe system, and we needed it quickly.

In 2001, we brought in General Motors consultants who introduced the PICOS methodology, an early Lean-based improvement process. GM had developed a "Program for the Improvement and Cost Optimization of Suppliers" (PICOS) to improve efficiency in their auto production, and we found the process itself could apply to our goals. Our first PICOS workshop focused on designing Unit 46, which, at that time, was the new Cardiology Unit where MAC and MATCS would be housed.

I'll never forget our first tough decision was whether to keep working on this—it was September 11, 2001. We kept working. The stakes were that high. We streamlined the process for admitting patients to the unit, standardized elements of the patient experience of care, and built reliable approaches to enable staff to do the work they loved.

Fast forward to 2004—our third PICOS workshop was co-facilitated by Shirley Weber, who was director of pathology and laboratory medicine then; Beth Clark, manager of Unit 46; and Terry Rusconi. There were 27 staff and leaders from nursing, laboratory, medical records, pharmacy, ER, admitting, perioperative, and IT all trying to figure out how to standardize best practices for the right information flowing to the right people. And we had needed an implementation plan to integrate and automate this clinical documentation system. Together, we created one.

From a cultural perspective, it was a watershed for us. We had received the warning from the TJC consultant in September or October, and in one week had our response. We showed folks across this relatively new organization what we were capable of and proved it to ourselves as well. Ultimately, we created what would become the foundation for our electronic medical record system, O^2: Optimal Outcomes. O^2 was a real-time, dynamic, multidisciplinary, automated record-keeping process that touched every part of the system.

We succeeded beyond our wildest dreams. And we proved the magnitude of what we could accomplish together.

Those wins helped us create the solid foundation that supports this organization, whether it's business as usual or a time of crisis.
—Tammy Peterman

Training and Measuring Progress

"We have high expectations of our people, and we want them to be successful," Bob Page said. Particularly when it comes to patient-first practice, "Employees can't be held accountable for something they don't know how to do," he pointed out. "We have to reinforce our vision with training."

From new employee orientation to ongoing professional development and education, KU Health System emphasized soft-skills training. The point was not just to increase awareness of what builds strong relationships but to use that awareness to measurably improve outcomes and the patient experience.

"Bob said he'd like to create a report every two weeks to be able to give all this data back to people," Paula Miller recalled. "Where are we succeeding and where are we not? It was all about transparency and reinforcement. I told him we could put it into an access database, and he said, 'Show me.' So I started the first customer satisfaction reports that we still use, although they've certainly been expanded."

LEADERSHIP LESSON:

Employees can't be held accountable for something they don't know how to do. You have to reinforce the vision with training to enable staff to be successful.

Telling Stories

Storytelling became the parlance of this culture—stories of KU Health System culture in action (see Chapter 9). Sharing what staff was doing right not only modeled the desired behavior, it celebrated the individuals and teams doing amazing work. It personalized the mission of this institution by providing real-life examples of what was expected of every staff member.

Stories are told not just to shine light on who's doing good things at The University of Kansas Health System, but to affirm to staff the crucial, direct influence it has on a patient's experience and outcomes.

"We want staff to know the tremendous impact they're having on our patients across this health system," says Tammy Peterman. "We want them to know they're moving the needle in the right direction."

Storytelling is the parlance of this culture. It personifies our mission and spotlights our culture in action. Sharing stories from the bedside up to the board room serves to teach, document, and celebrate our patients, our people, and our purpose.

Stories That Heal

Dear Every-Cancer-Patient-I-Ever-Took-Care-of,

I'm sorry. I didn't get it.

I've worked in oncology nearly my entire adult life. I prided myself in connecting with my patients and helping them manage their cancer. I really thought I knew what it's like to go through this. I didn't. I didn't get what it felt like to actually hear the diagnosis until I was hearing my own. I've been in on countless diagnosis conversations and had to give the news myself on plenty of occasions, but being "the person" the doctor is talking about is surreal. That day was the worst. I'm sorry. I didn't get it.

I didn't get how hard the waiting is—the diagnosis process takes forever. I didn't get how awkward it was to tell other people the news. You didn't know what to say. I didn't get how much you hung onto every word I said to you. Did I really mean this or that? You called me again to make sure. You asked your other nurses to see if you got the same answer. Please know we are happy to take a million calls a day with the same questions until you can make sense of it. I'm sorry. I didn't get it.

I didn't get how much you googled. I told you not to do it. But you did it, a lot—and so did I. I didn't get what it felt like to get the sad looks all the time. I didn't get how weird it felt to be called "brave." I didn't get why you were always suspicious. You couldn't help but wonder if we all knew something you didn't about your prognosis. You begged me for my input—to tell you what I would do if it were me. I hated that question, but I hear you now. I'm sorry. I didn't get it.

I didn't get how much you worried about your kids. For this, I'm the most regretful. I should've talked to you more about them, and not just in terms of lifting restrictions and germs.

I've probably had it a little easier than you—I know all these professionals and the vocabulary. I already know I'm in the best place I could be for treatment. I watched so many of you march through this terrible nightmare with a brave face and determination. You've always been my inspiration, and I love each and every one of you. Nothing brings me more joy than seeing you reach your goals and slowly put yourself back together. I love visits or notes from those of you who are several years out and doing great. It's good for a nurse's soul.

Even though healthcare workers don't really know what it's like to be you (well, us) it's okay. Nobody does. I just hope that I was still able to give you a little guidance and strength to help you get through your cancer treatment...even if I didn't get it.

Love,
Lindsay
—Lindsay Norris, KU Health System Oncology RN and Cancer Survivor,
2018 ANCC National Magnet Nurse of the Year
www.herecomesthesun927.com

The Culture Code

As the vision was upheld again and again in practice, the culture became codified with consistent expectations.

According to healthcare consultant and author Namita Seth Mohta, MD, "Change your organizational culture, and you change the patient experience."[8]

At KU Health System, that process was symbiotic. With every challenge met, the can-do zeitgeist gained momentum toward the vision. As the vision was upheld again and again in practice, the culture became codified with consistent expectations.

LEADERSHIP LESSON:

Our culture code melds philosophical values to organizational—and individual—behavior.

a. People come first, starting with patients and including employees.

- Focus on patients; when in doubt, do what's right for the patient.
- Cultivate an environment that promotes doing the right thing for the patient.
- Hire people who fit the culture and set them up for success.

b. Culture must be operationalized.

- Reinforce the vision and culture through training and ongoing communication.
- Use culture as strategy to inform systems and processes.
- Share stories that show this culture in action; shine the light on who's getting it right.

c. Ownership and outcomes must be transparent.

- Take responsibility for your part plus a little bit more so nothing is missed.
- Keep relevant, real-time data and make it accessible to everyone.
- Know your strengths and weaknesses; intervene accordingly.
- Be tough on systems, not people.

d. Collaboration and collegiality are SOP.

- Create multidisciplinary teams where everyone's input is expected and respected as standard operating procedure.
- Expect and support leadership at the bedside, not just in the executive offices.
- Lead by example from the top; you cannot delegate culture.
- Use consultants when necessary, but don't allow external input to compromise internal culture.

e. Successes get celebrated—whether incremental or meteoric.

- Celebrate, commemorate, and validate.
- Recognize and affirm the mission and vision in action.
- Be proud of what you've accomplished but never satisfied.

LEADERSHIP LESSON:

The culture code must be applied to hiring, training, observing, and measuring performance. Putting the patient first is not just an aspiration or advertising slogan, but an expectation with deliverables that staff knows how to meet.

This culture code was inculcated in training and practice, so patient-driven thinking was not an aspiration, but an expectation that staff knew how to meet. The culture generates a positive, ethically upright form of group-think that encourages consummate professionalism system-wide. It roots out defensiveness, arrogance, self-centrism, manipulation, and disrespect.

> The culture at KU Health System is upbeat. You get a sense that people like their jobs and like being here, which translates to better patient care and outcomes. From the housekeeper to the physician to the CEO, it is pervasive. If you pass executive leadership in the hall, they smile at you; they know your name. And I know the housekeeper's name, and the people I see in the cafeteria. People care about one another. It makes this a great place to work.
> —Jody Olson, MD

"It's the approachability and genuineness from everyone," said Jill Chadwick, media relations and MNN director at KU Health System. "I've seen a department director arrive late to a meeting because she took the time to walk a lost family member to a patient's room."

Cardiologist Charles Porter put it this way, "If you see the patient having some difficulty or if the room is just not quite right, you go out of your way to be sure the patient is taken care of. There are systematic 'random acts of kindness.' Somehow, they have that in every person who shows up here all the time, and that is really cool."

The culture generates a positive, ethically upright form of group-think that encourages consummate professionalism system-wide.

Innovation is encouraged as staff looks for compassionate ways to anticipate patient needs.

"We all get really creative with how to be helpful to patients," explained Kayla Northrop, RN. "Instead of thinking *that's not my job*, these efforts are supported and celebrated at KU Health System. When we bring the personalization, creativity, and care to patients beyond bed baths, meds, and treatments, we're helping them transition from being a victim to being a survivor.

"It's one thing to help someone heal from burns, but we want to heal the other aspects of the person that were injured," she added. "In fact, our vision statement that we created for this unit is *healing body, mind, and soul.* It's very holistic, and that approach is endorsed system-wide."

For KU Health System's Director of Patient and Family-Centered Services Rebecca Moburg, "The best way to describe this culture—and I hope everyone feels it when they walk in—is customer-centered."

Chief Culture Officer Terry Rusconi agreed, "We take this for granted, because it's normal for us, but one thing you will hear from people when they first come into the organization is 'something is different here.' They feel it the moment they walk in the door."

Ownership and Accountability

Imagine a team with almost 12,500 members sharing a goal that feels real and personal to each of them. When each member feels integral to its achievement on a personal level—while also feeling efficacy as part of a team—that's engagement. That kind of engagement directly impacts organizational performance.

"Employees want to believe their company has a meaningful purpose. They want to know that their own job is worthwhile. They want to make a difference. If all three of these conditions are accomplished, bottom-line results will follow."
—Quint Studer

Progress toward the goal must be transparent to every member of the team—even if there are nearly 12,500 of them.

"It was very important to hold ourselves measurably accountable, so everyone could see this was real and possible," Page said. "So organizational transparency was and continues to be essential."

Patient satisfaction is analyzed on everything from care to the facilities to the food and much more. Terry Rusconi was KU Health System director of performance improvement when he began overseeing the data collection and analysis with support from business intelligence developer Susan Graham. The analysis results in a kind of patient experience report card.

The results are reviewed every other Monday in leadership meetings that Page and Peterman first instituted in 1999. Tammy Peterman brings over 500 leaders from the Kansas City Division up to speed on current stats and relevant issues. Management takes the information back to the units and departments where recognition can be shared, improvements identified, and plans put into place to ensure continuous pursuit of excellence.

LEADERSHIP LESSON:

Acknowledge even small improvements. Setting a goal too high can be demoralizing to staff. Validating incremental progress creates many opportunities to affirm what's going right, which is a morale-booster.

The results weren't dazzling at first but, "We learned pretty quickly that we needed to acknowledge even small improvements," Page said. Page and Peterman realized it was important to recognize and celebrate whatever the data indicated was advancing.

Be Tough on Systems, Not People

KU Hospital's goal was unflinchingly measurable. But if units weren't hitting their goals, interventions focused on systems, not people. Even after a tragic medical error that resulted in the death of twin infants, the KUH mortality review team determined that the problem stemmed from a mistake in protocol, not human error.

"If that had been in any other hospital, someone or ones would have been fired," Bob Page said. "But that's not how we operate. What would we have learned from that tragedy if we scapegoated an employee who was just doing his job as directed? What would a decision like that do to the trust we've built with staff? You can't sustain a strong culture without trust."

Whether that means letting staff know how we are doing on key performance metrics or explaining a breakdown in care to a patient/family, transparency not only builds trust, it's critical to providing the best patient care.

"Early on, we were very transparent about our mistakes," acknowledged Tammy Peterman. "We've gone straight to the patient or family and said, 'We're sorry; we did this.' We sat in the room with an attorney whose mom was given the wrong medication with fatal results and said: *We are sorry*. When a family member died as a result of errors that occurred, we sat with those families and apologized."

Twenty years before it became a "best practice" in the industry, "We did this because it's our leadership philosophy and our culture—we own everything that's ours, including a mistake," Peterman said.

LEADERSHIP LESSON:

Transparency not only builds trust, it's essential to mistake-proofing the organization. If you own your mistakes and learn from them, you avoid making them again.

Improving the process is always the goal, and mistakes are gleaned for what can be learned. Tammy Peterman says, "We're tough on systems, not on employees."

As a result, the systems get stronger. And the proof is in the pudding. The operating room reached 100 days without "unintentionally retained foreign objects" by November 16, 2015. This was down from seven in six months the prior year thanks to an "*all-hands-on-deck* meeting called by system leadership in early August 2014," explained Liz Carlton, RN, vice president of quality and safety.

"We created the 'Chasing Zero' scorecard and focused on *zero harm* using raw numbers—not rates or percentages—with zero being the only acceptable result," she said. "Even though the rate might be phenomenal compared to other institutions or our own improvement, one patient being harmed is still one too many. Our OR was able to sustain zero unintentionally retained foreign objects for well over two years."[9]

HOW WE KNOW THAT

Leading by Example

Our culture works because it's lived at every level—from the board and executive office to the front lines of patient care and support. Tammy and I are routinely asked how we do this, because a lot of healthcare organizations are struggling with this issue. They want to know how we've pulled this off. I guess that means we're doing some things right! Here's part of the answer: lead by example.

I remember doing a workshop at another leading academic medical center on how to build a strong culture. We invited everyone there to introduce themselves and share his or her job title. After the last person spoke, Tammy and I just shook our heads in disbelief—not one person from senior executive leadership was in the group. We said, "Okay, this is not going to work. You can't delegate values; you can't assign culture to mid-management."

LEADERSHIP LESSON:

Leading by example means the expected behaviors start with the executive team. Your culture has to be modeled at the highest level. You can't delegate values or assign culture to mid-management.

In our culture, leadership means leading by example from the top. Tammy and I are marching rank and file with everyone else, working every single day to do the right thing for patients and achieve better outcomes. An executive's job is to ask, "What can I do to help you do your job better?"—not hand down decrees from on-high.
—Bob Page

The culture code of "mutual respect, honesty, loyalty, hard work—where all share the same goal at every level of the organization" extends system-wide, according to Marilyn Rymer. It manifests in the collegiality and collaboration of medical director partnerships, nursing leadership, multidisciplinary care teams, and countless other ways (see Chapter 5) that teamwork exemplifies the culture of KU Health System. Everyone's input is expected and respected—this is standard operating procedure.

Everyone's input is expected and respected—this is standard operating procedure at The University of Kansas Health System.

The People Who Come First

Pride in this culture is palpable. So, too, is the desire to protect it. When industry consultants are brought in to work on special projects, they don't last long if they don't understand and respect how the culture code works.

"The University of Kansas Health System probably has a stronger culture than anywhere else I've worked in terms of people being mission-driven and knowing why they're there," attested national healthcare consultant Chris Drummond of the Huron Consulting Group. "At our first meeting, I will tell you that Tammy Peterman was fairly cautious because she had so much pride in the culture, she didn't want anything to undo it."

Most consultants will say if you're spending 50 percent of your dollars on people, that's the area to start cutting. Tammy made it clear—we're not cutting people. That's not consistent with our culture.

Peterman's vigilance was uncompromised, especially when it came to any recommendation for tightening the budget by laying off employees.

"No matter who the consulting firm was, when they started talking about cost-savings, Tammy made it clear that we are not touching people," said Bob Page. "Most consultants will say if you're spending 50 percent of your dollars on people, that's the area to start cutting. Tammy made it clear—we're not cutting people. That's not consistent with our culture. People-first means patients, but it includes our own employees."

The Location Factor

Being in Kansas is an advantage in many important ways that aren't always obvious to outsiders.

Today, The University of Kansas Health System draws patients from every state in the nation and across the globe to this "fly-over" state.

"Being in Kansas is an advantage in many important ways that aren't always obvious to outsiders," said Wichita native Mark Uhlig, a KU Hospital Authority board member who spent years as a foreign correspondent for *The New York Times*. "I chose to come back to Kansas because I think the quality of the people and the community here are unequaled—the work ethic, the discipline, the honesty, and the highly educated workforce. The fact that it may sometimes be underestimated by outsiders just adds to its appeal, if you ask me."[10]

Prior to coming to KUH, I had interviewed with some prominent academic medical centers—those "you're lucky to get an interview" kinds of organizations. During the process, one of my colleagues recommended I talk with Bob Page. From the moment of our first interaction, I was struck by how different their recruitment approach was. It was the way recruitment should be done—the senior leaders taking a genuine interest in connecting with me on a personal level, helping me see how I would fit in, and showing me how I could have an impact. As I considered all the organizations where I was interviewing, it was clear that nothing compared to KUH. I knew I had to join their amazing team and be part of their incredible mission. I was hired as the chief human resources officer.

So I came to Kansas. Here's what I know now: I should have moved to the Midwest a long time ago. How people care for each other—their strong collaborative spirit and kindness—is a pervasive theme. Everyone in this hospital works together to do the right thing for patients every time—this is the guiding principle. I am trying to recruit my East Coast colleagues now!
—Julie Celano, KU Health System Senior Vice President and Chief Human Resources Officer, formerly with Brigham and Women's Hospital at Harvard Medical School

Those qualities factored heavily into the health system's response to the COVID-19 pandemic in the spring of 2020. According to TUKHS board member Doug Girod, MD, who is chancellor of the University of Kansas, the pandemic "presented massive challenges for the academic medical center campus, yet it also allowed rapid transformation in ways never thought possible—with long-term implications. They developed accelerated processes to design and implement clinical research trials, and they found their voice as leaders, locally, regionally, and nationally. Our AMC will forever be changed by the pandemic."

This achievement was possible because the people working within this organization were committed to their cultural values.

Julie Cerese, group senior vice president at Vizient, one of the nation's largest healthcare advisories, believes, "The University of Kansas Health System's greatest strength is a shared sense of purpose. The organization from top to bottom understands what it's trying to accomplish, and leadership is engaged in operations and supports others to align all these efforts."

Former KU Hospital Authority Board Chairman Greg Graves summed it up, "The University of Kansas Health System has made a science out of the art of culture. That has made all the difference for every person who comes here, as well as for the staff and service providers helping those patients and their families."

CHAPTER FOUR

Magnetize It

What you think, you become. What you feel, you attract.
What you imagine, you create.
—Buddha

Holly O'Brien had an idea. O'Brien, a nurse in the medical intensive care unit (MICU) was visiting with one of her patients, Megan, a young woman dying of cancer. Megan was hooked up to every machine possible and admitted that her biggest fear was that her daughter would be scared of her when she came to visit. So Holly had an idea. With Megan's permission, she took pictures of all the tubes and apparatus, then went home that night and "scrapbooked" the photos with easy-to-understand captions.

When Megan's little girl arrived, Holly read the book to her before she went into her mom's room. Holly explained how the ventilator was helping her mom breathe, and how the tubes were giving her mom medicine and nutrition. When they went into see Megan, this little girl was prepared. She saw her mama, not a room full of machines.

O'Brien's idea became *What's All This Stuff?*, a book that was used again and again, and later, with the family's permission, published for use in other organizations.

An Intentional Connection—Transforming the Hospital and Nursing

Nurses at The University of Kansas Health System are an amazing and remarkable team of highly engaged, well-educated, and totally invested professionals. They strive for improvement every day. They are motivated and motivational. They are learners and teachers.

These nurses are not only committed—they view what they do and how they do it as both a calling and a responsibility. Their work is a calling to advance evidence-based care and the practice of nursing, and a responsibility to patients, their peers, their profession, and the organization.

It is not an overstatement to say the transformation of The University of Kansas Hospital was directly correlated to the transformation of nursing.

Nursing as North Star

Saying patients come first, then actually ensuring the system works toward that goal, requires alignment of purpose and practice. Purpose was defined by the Five-Star Guiding Formula that became the navigation system for the hospital's transformation. But it was nursing that taught KUH how to put the formula into practice.

Nurses are the common denominator in all patient interactions. In the inpatient setting, nurses are with patients 24/7/365. And in the outpatient setting, they play a critical role in helping patients before, during, and after their visit. As The University of Kansas Hospital established quality performance measures for its Five-Star Guiding Formula, a clear understanding of the systems and processes resulting in an optimal patient experience was crucial. Nursing had the best vantage point.

"There is no better resource than our nursing staff for expertise in what it takes to provide patient-centered care," said Tammy Peterman.[1]

Patient outcomes provided objective data, but nurses brought insight that was often more timely and pragmatic. Through their skill, passion, knowledge, and focus on improvement, nursing became the "North Star" guiding the rest of the organization from formula into action.

If the Five-Star Guiding Formula was the navigation system, then it was nursing that taught KU Hospital how to put it into practice. Nursing became the North Star.

Aligning *purpose* and *practice* was critical to success. Yet one more element needed to be in place to fully achieve what the organization was being called to become. Nurses needed the authority to influence patient care and outcomes. In the late '90s, the hierarchy in the industry rarely supported such an obvious strategy.

"What we think of today as the practice of nursing was really non-existent back then," Jon Jackson noted.[2]

Doctors' orders were given priority because they referred patients to hospitals, and nurses were there to implement the orders written by the doctors.

Bob Page noted, "Ironically, 20 years ago, we didn't employ the physicians who were still contracted to KU's School of Medicine. But we did recruit, hire, orient, and support the nurses providing care to our patients."

> If you ask ten patients about their experience in the hospital, they'll all say they had wonderful care if they liked their nurse. Success is about having good doctors, there is no doubt, but without the same commitment from nurses—and to nursing—you aren't going to get there.
> —William A. Reed, MD

That direct connection to nursing was providential.

LEADERSHIP LESSON:

Nursing provides the best vantage point on patient-centric care. Nurses are the common denominator—the most consistent contact. The voice of nursing needs to be at every table where decisions get made about the planning and delivery of patient care—including in the board room. Nurses need the authority to influence patient care and outcomes.

"Nurses have more consistent and direct contact with patients—they are consistently involved in meeting the patient's needs," Peterman pointed out. Yet nursing leadership was marginalized or excluded, particularly at the executive level where patient care issues were discussed and decisions made. That was about to change at KU Hospital.

"I honestly couldn't believe any hospital could operate without the nurse executive as part of senior leadership," Page said. "One of the first things we did was to bring Tammy onto the senior leadership team."

It was a pivotal point in the hospital's transformation.

Peterman has reinforced the critical importance of nursing leadership. A practice she instituted and continued until moving to her system-level role was to interview the final candidates for nurse manager positions. For an organization as large as KU Health System, this was not standard practice. But it was important to Peterman for two reasons. The first was to ensure the culture fit and ability to lead the nursing organization forward. The second was to make sure these individuals knew how important the nurse manager role is and to know they'll get support from the executive levels of the organization.

Having a senior executive engaged at this level sends a powerful message about what the organization values and how the culture works. Even today, Peterman finds ways to stay connected to nursing leaders across all campuses. She understands what's going on at the bedside and in the boardroom.

Feel the Pull: Magnet® Designation as an Impetus for Better Patient Care

In 2001, Tammy Peterman was newly named chief nursing officer at KU Hospital. She believed *nurses must be autonomous in the practice of their discipline.* Patient satisfaction hinged on nursing care, so Peterman immediately focused on raising the level of professionalism, increasing the number of and support for nurses, and improving the image of nursing at KUH.

LEADERSHIP LESSON:

Just as there is a practice of medicine, there's a practice of nursing. Nurses must be autonomous in the practice of their discipline.

Peterman set her sights on a challenge: making The University of Kansas Hospital a Magnet® Hospital for Nursing Excellence. It would be the strongest commitment to and the ultimate credential for high-quality nursing.[3] For an institution that had been severely understaffed with high turnover rates among nurses only a few years earlier, this was an ambitious goal.

Peterman wasn't sure if they would get the designation, but "I knew we would be stronger because we were on the journey," she said.

The American Nurses Credentialing Center (ANCC) had developed the Magnet® designation in the early '90s to recognize an organization that consistently recruited and retained the best nurses. Those institutions that most embodied the "14 Forces of Magnetism" would be recognized as a Magnet® hospital. In the early years, candidates completed an exhaustive application process that documented ways in which they culturally exemplified the 14 "forces." To provide greater clarity and direction, as well as eliminate redundancy within the Forces of Magnetism, ANCC introduced an updated model that integrated the 14 Forces of Magnetism into 5 Model Components.[4] The new, simpler model reflected a greater focus on measuring outcomes and allowed for more streamlined documentation. Those Model Components are:

- Transformational Leadership
- Structural Empowerment
- Exemplary Professional Practice
- New Knowledge, Innovations, and Improvements
- Empirical Outcomes

To be a Magnet hospital was to be among the best of the best.

Bottom line: To be a Magnet hospital was to be among the best of the best. The Magnet journey would develop leaders within the nursing workforce and enhance relationships with other disciplines, but for Peterman, that wasn't the point.

"Those are important reasons, but not enough, not for us," Peterman explained. "If we have an engaged workforce, we have better outcomes for patients. So it begins with nursing, but it ultimately becomes a key element in achieving excellence in patient care. It's not about a trophy in the case, but a high-functioning, well-educated group of committed nurses who partner with physicians and other disciplines to provide the best care for patients. That is the endgame."

Bob Page attended the nursing retreat where Tammy Peterman and her staff began the Magnet conversation in earnest.

"Tammy empowered the nursing staff to come up with their own nursing vision statement," he said. "It was important for it not to be coming from the executive office."

At the retreat, during follow-up focus groups, and by reaching out to every nurse for input and feedback hospital-wide, a vision emerged: *Taking pride in our practice, The University of Kansas Hospital nurses lead the way, merging science with compassion in delivery of exceptional patient care.*

The nurse-driven visioning process, successful at an organizational level, proved equally invaluable in creating a sense of ownership and commitment as it cascaded to each specialized unit, serving as the foundation for unique, unit-level visions.

"From all those discussions, the nursing staff came up with a customized vision statement for their own unit," Peterman said.

The growing sense of self-determination bolstered by executive support would leverage nursing into new realms of influence.

HOW WE KNOW THAT

Nursing Defines the Model of Care

I remember standing in front of one of our leadership team meetings announcing nursing would own patient satisfaction. While I knew nursing couldn't fix everything that was broken, I did know if nurses were supported to provide exceptional care, the patient experience would be enhanced. I then told all the leaders outside of the division of nursing their job was to ensure nursing had what they needed to achieve the highest levels of patient satisfaction—to partner with and support them in every way possible.

This singular change in "ownership" began to shift the dial. Every nurse in this hospital is a leader, and this change affirmed that principle. We empower and authorize nurses to innovate, create, and lead. Now we were saying *the organization is going to back you in those efforts.* Everyone is here to support you and will work with you to fix what isn't working in our existing systems and processes.

This singular change in "ownership" began to shift the dial. Every nurse in this hospital is a leader, and this change acknowledged it.

Fast forward to today. People want to work here. Pandemic aside, we normally have two to three times the nursing applications than we have open positions. Even during recent nursing shortages, we have not faced the challenge of not being able to fill our positions with competent, capable, passionate, and engaged staff. The goal established by the Institute of Medicine in its *The Future of Nursing* report is to have 80 percent of the bedside nurses holding baccalaureate degrees by the year 2020. Well, we already had over 80 percent in our hospital by 2017 and were over 88 percent as 2020 came to a close.

When we round on staff, that commitment to patient care is obvious. We ask what creates the most pride for them, and the number-one answer is the team they work with. They also talk about the ability to provide great care to patients and the outcomes they are generating. And they tell us they want to stay here, knowing they have many career opportunities spanning bedside care, education, research, information technology, and leadership.

> Everything we do to improve nursing care will improve outcomes for patients. In my opinion, nursing will define the future model of success for our entire industry.
> —Bob Page

The Magnet Journey

Tammy Peterman and Suzanne Shaffer, RN, began the formal Magnet® application process in 2002.

"Good nursing care was being provided for patients, but Magnet gave us an opportunity to focus on everything we could do to improve on that," Peterman emphasized. "Magnet became the blueprint to raise the level of professionalism and practice, and to provide the best practice environment for nurses. Ultimately, that would have a huge impact on patients."

Since the Magnet review would consider all aspects of nursing, KU Hospital would, too.

Peterman explained, "Magnet looks at everything…teamwork on the unit—are physicians and nurses working well together? Do nurses have the resources they need? Are nurses valued? Are education and continuing professional development for nurses supported and encouraged? Is there strong leadership in nursing across the organization?"

The Magnet committee developed their metrics for high performance based on all 14 Forces of Magnetism. No stone was left unturned when looking to codify excellence in every form and facet of nursing care.

LEADERSHIP LESSON:

The process of achieving Magnet® designation became the blueprint to raise the levels of professionalism and practice, and to enhance nursing's reputation and image. Ultimately, that had a huge impact on patients.

Internal surveys were done to assess engagement. The results indicated nurses perceived themselves as providing high-quality care to their patients and viewed high-quality care as a hospital priority. This was a good start, but there was so much more to be done.

Every nurse is a leader through the work they do. Formalizing that leadership capacity through a strong and vibrant council structure would prove instrumental in advancing the Magnet® journey. The first nursing councils were convened to assess, analyze, and evaluate clinical and operational processes and outcomes as a direct expression of their new authority.

These councils took ownership of ensuring high-quality care across the organization by immersing themselves in the available data: monitoring patient satisfaction surveys, understanding and addressing regulatory standards, enabling optimal documentation compliance, and improving performance on quality indicators. They focused on key indicators linked to the organizational goals, including mortality, patient safety (falls, restraint usage, adverse medication events), pressure ulcer incidence and prevalence, hospital-acquired infections, pain management, and more.

Nursing leadership produced new, more inclusive policies, protocols, and communication structures. Like never before, nurses were contributing to the science and evidence of patient care through nursing-led research studies. Nurses had designated roles on collaborative decision-making teams with doctors, pharmacists, and hospital management.

The clinical assessment by nurses was not only valued, it was requested as they became fully-integrated members of the team. The old-school medical hierarchy with doctors at the top of the pyramid shifted to multidisciplinary dialogues where everyone's input was expected and respected, and reliant on the voice of nursing.

There was such a strong sense of teamwork. It was exciting.

Nancy Martin, RN, had already been at KU Hospital for 29 years when she became chair of the newly formed Nursing Clinical Practice Council in 2005.

"It was both scary and inspiring," she said. "Now we had all these nurse representatives coming together to talk about the great things they were doing and what their challenges were. We talked about the projects that were underway in the units to help provide better care for the patients. We explored ways we could help other units. There was such a strong sense of teamwork. It was exciting."

Consistent and collegial communication between nurses and doctors, as well as other members of every healthcare team, became standard operating procedure. The hospital committed adequate staff for the work environment. Data related to improving patient satisfaction and patient outcomes was collected by nurses for the hospital's performance improvement initiatives. The information helped identify and objectify problems, as well as show improvement trends or areas in need. Solutions were discussed as a multidisciplinary team, so every element of the issue could be explored and all were invested in the process.

According to Terry Rusconi, who was director of organizational development at the time, "It wasn't just physicians leading the dialogue. There were nurse managers and other managers across the organization working in partnership to improve outcomes."

> Nurses own patient satisfaction? This was a new way of thinking for most of us. Many of the issues were rooted in housekeeping, food service, and other areas. What could we, as nurses, do about the issues felt to be out of our control? But once nurses knew the executive leadership was going to support them, they began to engage and problem-solve with the other departments. New policies were put into place hospital-wide that wouldn't allow bullying: nurse-to-nurse, physician-to-nurse, etc. We committed to a zero-tolerance policy about that. Nurses felt increasing trust in the process. We began to see we were being supported, not just called out to blame when things went wrong. On the shared decision-making councils that now included staff nurses, we realized nurses weren't alone in finding the solutions.
> —Suzanne Shaffer, RN

In 2006, KU Hospital's application was ready for the Magnet® review, and by then everyone had a stake in the result.

"We orchestrated the route of the cars driving the appraisers to the campus," Terry Rusconi recalled. "They went by Westwood, where the accounting and other staff were on the curb welcoming them and celebrating the Magnet site visit. We also had folks at key intersections along the route to ensure the appraisers could begin to feel the importance of nursing across the organization. It was all to demonstrate the cross-disciplinary commitment to this important accreditation—everyone from EVS to executive team members were proud to participate in the early morning welcoming event."

No nursing unit could earn this award on its own merits, alone. This was about our whole team. It was driven by the spirit and culture we have here.

Achieving Magnet® designation would put The University of Kansas Hospital in an exclusive field. There were only 200 Magnet hospitals in the nation at that time. Magnet recognition is earned by only 7 percent of the nation's 6,000 hospitals.[5] After a four-year journey toward the goal, KU Hospital received its first Magnet® designation the first time it applied in 2006. It maintained this status through the next two review cycles in 2011 and 2016. Only 3.9 percent of the nation's hospitals earn the designation three times or more in a row.[6]

For Nancy Martin, RN, who retired in 2017, the achievement was the pride of her 41-year career.

"It means we are among the best across the country," she said. "No hospital nursing unit could receive this recognition on its own merits, alone. This was about our whole team. It was driven by the spirit and culture we have here."

The Pedagogy of Care

The Magnet journey transformed nursing at KU Hospital. Chris Ruder, RN, was a nursing director in those days.

"It was a new era, but there were still the same number of hours in a day," said Ruder, who would go on to become COO of KU Health System's Kansas City Division. "We often felt rushed. Like everybody else in healthcare, we felt like we never had enough time. But that whole 'busy' demeanor can be a barrier."

And barriers had to come down.

"When our patients and their families heard us ask, 'What else can I do for you? What else can I get for you? I have the time,' it let them know they were the most important thing on our minds—because they were, and they still are," added Ruder. "It says, I am not thinking about the next patient or the next situation; I'm focused on your needs. Putting it in the official 'script' gave staff permission to take the time to genuinely be there. So I think there is this concept of being mindful and present."

Always a Better Way

Today, nurses are writing their own articles, doing research, and developing training curriculums for directing and delivering patient care. Innovation in all aspects of nursing is encouraged at KU Health System, as is learning of best practices that can be adapted for use in a particular setting or across the organization. If a protocol or procedure can be made more efficient or effective, it should be, and nurses are expected to design, test, and implement new ideas as part of their daily work.

Tori Butler, RN, former nurse manager in medical telemetry, described why a fresh approach to dispensing medications in her unit was needed.

"The process had been very robotic and passive for patients," she recalled. "They had a medication due, then the nurse came in, followed policy on the seven-rights-of-medication administration. Then, when giving the medication, the nurse would either tell them what they were taking or just say, 'Here is your morning medicine, Mrs. Smith.' With this process, we were not assessing the patient's understanding of the medication, nor were we providing and reinforcing education of that medication or its side effects. The patients in these situations were passive in their care. Then at discharge they would get a bolus of education—which was not optimal."

LEADERSHIP LESSON:

If a protocol or procedure can be made more efficient or effective, it should be, and nurses can initiate a new approach.

Perhaps this wasn't a pressing issue that called for immediate corrective action—but for an organization committed to putting the patient at the center of care, it wasn't setting the patient up for success upon discharge. Butler's team knew they could do better.

"We shifted our focus to make the patient a more active participant and learner in his or her own care," she explained. "We would do the medication pass utilizing the teach-back methodology, while also assessing their level of understanding. We'd say, 'Good morning, Mrs. Smith, I have your pills for this morning. Tell me what pills you usually take with breakfast.'

"This allowed the nurse to assess the patient's understanding of his or her medication," said Butler. "Then, if the patient was able to correctly tell us what he or she takes, we discussed side effects. If he or she did not know, then we provided education—printed written information—and placed it in a binder to take home at discharge. At each medication pass, this was done, which supported and reinforced that learning."

LEADERSHIP LESSON:

Processes that are routine and robotic are not going to meaningfully engage patients. Nurses can shift patients from passive to active roles with innovative, personal interactions. That results in patients who are better prepared to return home and maintain the right self-care to stay out of the hospital.

Part and parcel to this was the ongoing data collection that would indicate whether the new process was working.

"The patient satisfaction surveys showed a great increase in the patients' understanding of medication, and we also started to see a decrease in the readmission of patients to the hospital," Butler said, adding that the feedback indicated "the patients loved the education binders we created with them and the time we took to educate them."

The Rise of Nursing Leadership

Today, bedside nurses, unit educators, clinical nurse specialists, and frontline staff are all champions for the zero-harm initiatives at The University of Kansas Health System. Their firsthand insight into patient risks uniquely positions them to come up with practical, feasible solutions or (just as valuable) to recognize ideas that weren't really workable and offer alternatives.

> Before I came to KU, I worked in outpatient mental health. I brought my office mate's client here—he had such challenges including mental illness, illiteracy, homelessness, and a cancer diagnosis. They treated my friend John with such compassion and kindness… everyone was so nice in helping me find resources for him.
>
> So I fell in love with this hospital before I fell in love with nursing. But that experience made me want to be a nurse—I mean I wanted to be a nurse tomorrow! It still works like that here—this place is magical.
> —Miki Mahnke, RN, BSN, CMSRN, Nurse Manager

Unit Educator Janet Marts, RN, BSN, MSN, PCCN, affirms, "The suggestions from the bedside staff are taken seriously, and those ideas are often implemented. If the quality team thinks a practice change would work to decrease hospital-acquired conditions, but the bedside staff does not feel it's practical or useful, that feedback is taken seriously. The bedside staff feel they have a voice about the care they deliver. That is something I did not see at other hospitals where I've worked."

LEADERSHIP LESSON:

If the bedside staff doesn't think a new idea or practice change is realistic or effective, that carries a lot of weight. Leadership at the bedside is exactly that—pragmatic leadership.

In 2011, another nursing role was introduced. The position of "nurse navigator" was implemented to help patients, their families, and advocates "navigate" their way through what, for them, were uncharted waters. Nurse navigators help ensure all of the needed documents are collected and prepared for the medical team, and appointments are scheduled in a timely manner with the appropriate care team members. The popularity of nurse navigators has prompted expansion of this program.

When my dad was diagnosed with cancer, I would have really benefited from a checklist of tips and resources designed for the caregiver, not the patient. I needed help. So when the opportunity came for us to help KU Health System philanthropically, we sat down with wonderful doctors and nurses and discussed the feelings I had about that experience and how we could improve. We came up with the wonderful "nurse navigator" program for the Cancer Center. It was what we were lacking when I felt so lost.

The nurses and doctors involved with this are the most dedicated people I've seen as far as taking a concept and following through—crossing every *t* and dotting every *i*. Now there's a nurse navigator who holds your hand all the way through the patient process. It's quite comforting and it's much more efficient.

We actually then went through this personally when I was here for cancer treatment myself. In fact, I was actually the first person to receive the navigator book that we had been working on. It was terrific.[7]
—Teresa Walsh

Nurse-Initiated Improvements Grow Future Leaders

Nurse-led research is another expanding function. One innovative study on alternative therapies for pain mediation done by KU Health System nurses made national news in 2017. It was designed to decrease narcotic use while improving patients' comfort and decreasing pain, anxiety, and nausea.

Lead author Megan Moore, RN, said, "Being given the opportunity and support to implement research as a nurse at The University of Kansas Health System has allowed us to provide a way to individualize patient needs. We're empowered to look outside of the box, and that is exactly what we did. We explored non-pharmacological approaches because of the danger of opioid over-prescription.

"Our measures have provided a profound amount of comfort to our patients," she added. "As the nurses behind this research, the encouragement to be creative in meeting our patients' needs and seeing the phenomenal impact of this effort drives us to want to do more and more for the patients we serve."

As the nurses behind this research, the encouragement to be creative in meeting our patients' needs and seeing the phenomenal impact of this effort drives us to want to do more and more for the patients we serve.

Optimizing Best Practices

The comprehensive patient rapid response model was initially inspired by an Institute for Healthcare Improvement (IHI) conference in 2004. Peterman, Page, and a group from KU Hospital came back with a plan for implementing "rapid response teams," one of six best practice initiatives included in IHI's "100,000 Lives Campaign" to prevent avoidable deaths from medication errors, lack of standard care for heart attack patients, or preventable infections.

Bob Page said, "We implemented RRTs in very short order. When patients are the focus of your operation, you can do that."

Casey Pickering, RN, nurse manager of the MICU and program manager for the rapid response and code blue program, added, "We were one of the first in the country to implement a rapid response team to deploy to any medical emergency across the entire campus, not just in the inpatient setting."[8]

LEADERSHIP LESSON:

We implemented rapid response teams in very short order. That kind of agility is possible only when everybody's got their eyes on the same goal: doing what's right for patients.

At first, the goal of the rapid response team (RRT) was to get an expert critical care team consisting of an ICU nurse and a respiratory therapist at a patient's bedside to intervene appropriately and early. There were 20 activations in the first month, but as awareness of the RRT grew, use of the resource did, too. After the first year, the survival rate for RRT activations was 78 percent. Being able to get those additional resources to the bedside earlier created a vast improvement over the 10 percent national average for code blue survival at the time.[9]

"We now have 24/7 dedicated effort for rapid response and code blue coverage, in addition to the staff who respond from the various ICUs," Pickering said.

By 2018, the team averaged 320 activations per month, and patient survival rate for RRT activations had increased to 90.7 percent.[10]

"When the team was implemented, they covered the single, original hospital building," Pickering said. "Our organization has grown considerably since then to include the Heart Center and Cambridge Tower. Our team expanded as the demand nearly tripled and as our footprint expanded. We brought on additional staff from several other ICUs to help with team coverage."

Today, the RRT model continues to be deployed as originally designed. And the success of the RRT model has further expanded to provide additional resources in a wide variety of settings. Targeted response teams have been created for stroke, code blue, trauma, burns, E-STAT (emergently to the operating room), code neo (imminent delivery), behavior, patient safety events, sepsis, and STEMI (ST-elevation myocardial infarction/cardiac). Each team includes bedside nurses and healthcare providers from all relevant areas who have the skills and knowledge to support the staff and ensure optimal patient outcomes.

LEADERSHIP LESSON:

Rapid response teams focused on specific patient needs are the hallmark of our model. The specializations vary from code blue to code neo to behavior concerns and more. And anyone—including a patient's family member—can call in a concern to activate the patient safety response team.

Response teams focused on specific needs are the hallmark of the KU Health System Model. Case in point, the patient safety response team (PSRT) can be activated by anyone (including a family member) who has either been part of or is concerned about the potential for a serious safety event that could harm a patient or the system.

An internal call to 588-SAFE can be placed any time day or night. The hotline is staffed by one of the risk coordinators—each is a nurse and a member of the patient safety response team. The risk coordinator gathers information and assesses the severity and potential risk of the situation. Those that have resulted in or have the potential for causing harm result in the activation of the PSRT. The team meets virtually or on site to mitigate a problem or intervene if harm has occurred. It provides support to patients, families, and staff, and is responsible for ensuring processes have been put into place to keep the identified issue from causing future harm.

LEADERSHIP LESSON:

When a crisis arises, immediate interventions are put in place to ensure the safest care and no further harm occurs. Next is to make sure the problem or error doesn't travel—that is, to keep it from happening anywhere else in the system. Finally, make sure staff is okay. Being involved in a patient safety response crisis can be traumatizing, so resources are in place to also meet staff needs.

Nurse Residency Program Features an Escape Room for Nurses

In 2003, The University of Kansas Hospital was one of the first in the country to join with University HealthSystem Consortium to introduce a formal nurse residency program (NRP). Six years later, the health system became one of the first post-baccalaureate NRPs in the nation to be accredited by the Commission on Collegiate Nursing Education.

The NRP provides education and support for the new nurse over an entire year. In addition to unit orientation, new nurses also attended monthly NRP seminars. The seminars focused on education and support to the new graduate.

"When we started, our format was very similar to nursing school," explained Robyn Setter, MS, RN, who helps coordinate the program. "There were lectures for two hours and then small group time with a facilitator to work on unit education, discuss issues, and work on projects. This has morphed over the last 15 years, and we now have interactive seminars ranging from stations to learn different aspects of a topic to the escape room at the end of the year."[11]

The first year there were 51 new graduates, Setter said of the nurse residency program. Fifteen years later, 2,350 individuals have completed the NRP. From the beginning, the average overall first-year retention rate has remained at 94 percent.

Director of Quality and Safety Amanda Gartner, RN, was among the first NRP graduates.

"Over the past several years, I have seen a significant transformation in the content, effectiveness, and utility of this program for our new graduate nurses," says Gartner. "The first year of nursing is overwhelming—this program offers a venue for critically important peer support and a safe environment for coping and learning," she said. "The program also provides an opportunity for these nurses to get involved in meaningful quality improvement and patient safety projects."

The "escape room" experience was created as a way to integrate gaming technology and adult learning principles. The nurse residents used information they had received during their residency and on the unit over the course of the year to solve the challenge and escape each room. Those challenges included:

- Putting a nine-piece puzzle together, which revealed a medication calculation they had to solve to receive the next clue;
- Correctly identifying a patient using dual identifiers prior to administering a medication;
- Using their knowledge of pressure injuries to identify and accurately stage four pressure injuries;
- Identifying the items found in the "Fall Prevention Backpack" revealed after the previous step;
- Identifying the current patient safety goals; and
- Identifying and incorporating SBAR (situation, background, assessment, recommendation). Nurse residents were asked to participate in the experience to help demonstrate their knowledge and understanding of the learning objectives of the nurse residency program.

The first objective of this experience was to change the format of how nurses are trained from a passive approach, with lecture and slides, to an active learning approach incorporating game-based learning. The second objective was to evaluate if nurse residents retained the information received during the yearlong residency seminars. This was measured during the interactive escape room activity.

Ninety-five percent of participating nurse residents felt confident they were performing skills accurately, and 91 percent felt the activity provided an opportunity to demonstrate their knowledge. Survey responses were positive—for example: "It was awesome: such a fun, unique way to apply hospital policies and procedures" and "It makes you realize it's important to pay attention to small details."

In March 2017, the residency coordinators shared the escape room concept at the Vizient/American Association of Colleges of Nursing Conference, and in 2018 presented information on how to create an escape room to over 1,600 nurses at the ANCC National Magnet Conference. This unique training tool has since been replicated in hospitals in 48 states and internationally.[12]

The North Star Shines on the Bedside

Over the course of time, stories from the bedside have both celebrated the paths nurses have walked to make a difference for their patients and lit the way for others to follow. There are no policies to tell people how to go that extra mile, just the expectation Bob Page sets with every new employee: "If you make the decision that's right for the patient, you will never make a wrong decision."

While excited about a long-anticipated organ transplant, Valentin was conflicted. His plan to take the Oath of Allegiance to become a U.S. citizen earlier in the spring of 2020 was derailed by cardiac complications that resulted in his hospitalization. His nursing team, Kathleen Sullivan, Emma Schelble, and Anna Fisk, could hear how disappointed Valentin was. They personally reached out to a federal judge, explained the situation, and asked if he could help. On April 8, the judge came to the hospital, and in the Bell Sanctuary inside the foyer, the Oath of Allegiance was administered with Valentin's family and staff present to celebrate his citizenship (including a cookie cake).

That approach has inspired many great moments in TUKHS nursing.

Nurse Manager Rebecca Ramel, RN, recalled her unit's innovation with a patient who had a traumatic brain injury that manifested in difficult behavior.

"It was very hard to manage when we first admitted her," Ramel said. "She had frequent behavioral outbursts and aggression toward staff. The team worked with her to develop a daily schedule and a reward system for good behavior. She began to thrive with the structure and the relationships she was building with our team.

"The patient was in the hospital for an extended period of time and often expressed to the nursing staff a desire to work, specifically doing secretarial-type tasks," added Ramel. "The team created a job for her in her hospital room, mostly cutting pictures and letters out of paper. We made fake money and paid her for her time, then at the end of every week she would get to go shopping in a fake store we created in my office. Most of the items were donated by staff, things she needed like shampoo, but also things she loved liked lip gloss and nail polish. A few of the nurses came in one evening on their day off and took her out for a picnic on hospital grounds, bringing her favorite foods."

The team truly embraced this patient and found a creative way to manage her behavior and make her long hospital stay enjoyable for her. A few of the nurses came in one evening on their day off and took her out for a picnic on hospital grounds, bringing her favorite foods.

A Culture That Creates Shining Stars

Magnet® recognition was an important achievement, but it was not the end goal. From the start, the real value to the organization was in the blueprint it provided—a blueprint the organization personalized and embedded in the culture already being developed.

Tammy Peterman points out the big picture is even "bigger than nursing. Magnet designation is very nursing-specific. However, consistent with our patient-centered and team-based culture, we wanted the entire organization to embrace the foundational principles of Magnet. Every effort in all departments and service lines is aligned to fully meet or exceed patient needs."

Transplant surgeon Sean Kumer said, "I round early in the morning and we have daily group huddles—nurses are integral to both. We have meetings every day to make sure we're dealing with problems that come up or could come up. Collaboratively, we plan for the day, the week, or the month—whatever's necessary. We talk about each patient's individual situation as a multidisciplinary team. Then someone from this team who was part of that conversation goes on to meet with another unit where that patient will be moved."

Every effort in all departments and service lines is aligned to fully meet or exceed patient needs.

That collegiality and cooperation is standard operating procedure across campus. Gail Schuetz, assistant inpatient CNO, put it this way, "I feel like we became a close-knit family and somehow we've been able to keep that feel despite massive growth."

Peterman and Page would say that's about KU Health System's culture.

No opportunity is missed to spotlight nursing achievements.

The University of Kansas Health System culture is expressed in the many ways nursing excellence is recognized. From the Health System Magnet Nurse of the Year, to every type of DAISY Award available, to donor-supported awards and nursing excellence awards and so much more, recognition is part of the organizational DNA.

No opportunity is missed to spotlight nursing achievements. Units with the highest levels of patient satisfaction are acknowledged. Whenever a patient references a nurse by name via feedback on "KU Care Cards," that nurse is commended within his or her unit as well and word makes it to the executive team. Nurses are often invited to board meetings to be recognized. During Nurses' Week and other special events, additional recognition for outstanding daily work can include free drinks in the cafeteria, gift certificates to area restaurants, department stores, free movie passes, and tickets to sporting events.

The Best Nursing in the Nation

The American Nurses Credentialing Center presents the annual National Magnet Nurse of the Year Awards to five clinical nurses working at Magnet-designated hospitals from across the nation. Recipients at The University of Kansas Health System include:

Melanie H. Simpson, PhD, RN-BC, OCN, CHPN, coordinator of the Pain Management Resource Center, in 2012. Simpson helped form the pain management team at KU Hospital in 2001, and the Coalition for Comprehensive Pain Management, in which hospital clinicians and representatives from The University of Kansas Medical Center's three schools convene quarterly to discuss the latest evidence-based pain management research.

Debbie Pennington, RN, BSN, in 2014, for creating the nation's first Neonatal Medical Home. Annually, the clinic sees about 700 unique patients from birth through age five, most of them "graduates" from the NICU. The clinic's staff is a single point of contact for these medically complex children.

Lindsay Norris, RN, in 2018, in recognition of her ongoing education of health system staff, health professionals, and members of the public across the country and the world. That education began with a simple blog. Her inspiration to better educate and equip her teams comes from a personal battle with Stage 3 colorectal cancer that began in 2016. Lindsay's blog has been translated into at least four languages, been viewed by over one million people, and is used in multiple healthcare programs to help teach empathy.

LEADERSHIP LESSON:

Magnet is a blueprint. The value of that blueprint is visible in what patients experience, the team feels, and the appraisers see. What they see is a group of nurses and staff who love what they do, love who they work with, and love the organization in which they work.

HOW WE KNOW THAT

What You Imagine, You Create—a Great Hospital with Great Nurses Now and into the Future

This chapter begins with a powerful quote about imagination. When we began our Magnet® journey in 2002, we imagined an organization where the practice of nursing was strong and well respected, where the image of nursing was of a trusted, professional colleague. We imagined a place in which nurses—respected for their independent thinking, exemplary practice, and collaborative approach—truly became partners with physicians and other clinicians.

We imagined an environment where nurses would share what they had learned and discovered as best practices across the metro, the region, and the nation. We imagined being an academic medical center known as a local, regional, and national leader, a source of new knowledge and best practices that transformed patient care. And we dreamt of being a place where nurses (and others) were drawn because they knew it was an exceptional environment for providing care and creating great outcomes.

All of what we had imagined in our Magnet® journey has been achieved, and more. We know that from data showing our outcomes for patients, our patient satisfaction ratings, our nursing retention rates and engagement scores, and the increased volume of patients we serve. We know that from feedback from physicians and stories from patients.

However, we are an organization that is "proud but never satisfied." That's part of what makes us different. We could have said we'd checked everything off that list; let's take a break. Instead, we know there's more to do. Future nurses, physicians, and other healthcare professionals will engage in writing the next chapters of patient care.

Our faithfulness to and personalization of the Magnet model has reinforced the culture we set out to create. It's provided a strong foundation on which to build. Most importantly, we have established a system that doesn't rely on Bob or me to be sustained into the future. We are the current guardians of that system. Our job as leaders is to help grow the next generation of guardians who will imagine an even greater organization than the one we have today.
—Tammy Peterman

Magnet is a blueprint. The value of that blueprint is visible in what the patients experience, the team feels, and the appraisers see. Peterman attests, "What they see is a group of nurses and staff who love what they do, love who they work with, and love the organization in which they work."

CHAPTER FIVE

Question It

By doubting we are led to question,
and by questioning we arrive at the truth.
—Peter Abelard

Ironically, it was the day before Valentine's Day in 2019, a random detail Beth Eide, RN, remembered clearly about this particular "red event." It might have been just another day at the office for some...except at The University of Kansas Health System, it wasn't.

As with all safety intelligence (SI) reports she received as risk manager, Eide's first question was whether the patient involved had suffered any harm. Britany Leiker, RN, who submitted the SI report, was clear: The patient was okay. Amanda Gartner, director of quality & safety, had the same concern when she read the report. Gartner alerted Quality Outcomes Coordinator Lauren Eck, RN, who, along with Danielle Young, RN, would coordinate the escalation of the issue via the patient safety response team (PSRT).

The SI report indicated that a pump dispensing drugs intravenously went "free flow," so all the medication was delivered in 30 minutes instead of via a regulated drip-feed over several hours. Thanks to quick mitigation by the medical team, the patient suffered no adverse reactions. That part was known and stabilized, but the full-court press was now bearing down on what had caused this. The PSRT had already been convened for a mobile conference call with reps from pharmacy, risk management, executive leadership, and the equipment vendor.

Intention and Inquisition

When lives are at risk, the right response depends on people as much as protocols. "If you have compassion for patients, you may be more meticulous about somebody's care, have higher quality standards, and be less prone to making medical errors," says Stephen Trzeciak, MD, MPH, coauthor of *Compassionomics*.[1]

In this case, and in every case, the people bringing the right intentions to the rapid response process demonstrate KU Health System's culture in action. It's a culture that invokes autonomy in each individual within an infrastructure of collaboration. The net result is a holistic, multi-faceted focus on the patient from every operational perspective.

It's a culture that invokes autonomy in each individual within an infrastructure of collaboration. The net result is a holistic, multi-faceted focus on the patient from every operational perspective.

With multi-disciplinary rigor, the review began. User error was ruled out by cross-checking with electronic pharmacy data, but two other SI reports citing suspicious flow issues surfaced.

"We began to tie that all together," Beth Eide explained.

The matter was elevated to the level of "red event," and the SI report was on Justin Schmidt's desk within 24 hours. Schmidt, KU Health System's regulatory and accreditation coordinator at that time, was only too familiar with what needed to happen next.

Sweating the Small Stuff

Every day in hospitals nationwide, patient safety issues and equipment problems of all kinds increase the stress on systems. On any given day, about 1 in 31 hospital patients has at least one healthcare-associated infection.[2] KU Health System's exhaustive focus on "zero harm" is addressing that trend.

"I think the difference for us is that we question our process until it's pinned to the mat—we are fixated on the fix," said Bob Page.

That inquisitional process is how Schmidt discovered tubing was the issue in 2019—and not just for Leiker. Morgan Whisenhunt, RN, also submitted an SI report about the same problem.

"SI concerns are thoroughly investigated," assured Schmidt. "Those reports can make a difference, not only at our health system, but, as in these cases, to other hospitals nationwide."

Safety incident reports can make a difference, not only at our health system, but, as in these cases that led to FDA recalls, to healthcare nationwide.

Leiker and Whisenhunt had red-flagged a serious problem that would ultimately result in a national product recall of more than 25,000 defective PCA infusion sets from hospitals around the country in May 2019.[3]

That same month, thanks to due diligence by the PSRT, along with Justin Schmidt's scrutiny that alerted the healthcare industry at large to the problem, an entire fleet of faulty IV pumps were FDA recalled. The recall ranked among the nation's largest for medical equipment, with more than 150 million devices involved.[4] The U.S. Food and Drug Administration even issued a certificate praising The University of Kansas Health System's "outstanding contribution in promoting patient safety with medical devices."

LEADERSHIP LESSON:

We encourage everyone on staff to question anything that is a barrier to care, and the employee who noticed must be authorized to handle it...but no one has to handle it alone. As leaders, it's our job to make sure every employee feels the "we've got your back" assurance within this culture.

"We encourage everyone on staff to question anything that is a barrier to care, but no one has to handle it alone," Tammy Peterman said. "As a unit, as managers, and as an organization, we want every employee to feel the 'we've got your back' assurance of this culture."

And feel it they do.

In fact, incidents that began by a patient's bedside "have impacted the nation because our staff brought them through our escalation channels," Amanda Gartner said. "Our staff feels safe escalating concerns when they're taking care of patients in this environment."

Not just safe, but empowered.

Medical Assistant Jessie King carefully checked every piece of equipment that would be needed in the examination room. That was standard operating procedure, but this time she noticed something substandard. One of the scopes had passed only two of the three required checks she did before every single sterile procedure. Two out of three would not clear the bar...not here—not on Jessie King's watch. King stopped the line, pulled the scope, and alerted the manager. Nothing would go forward until she replaced the scope and reset the room. It took extra time and attention, but King wasn't going to take the risk.

"It's so important that she felt comfortable doing that," said Senior Director of Nursing Gloria Solis, RN. "It can be hard to tell docs and authority figures, 'Hey, we're going to be late but we're doing it right,' when you're the support staff, but Jessie felt comfortable doing that and so she did. All of our patients deserve professionals like Jessie."

Today, the message is, *If safety even tickles your mind, call.* Staff is not only encouraged but expected to report safety concerns—despite who's involved and what happened.

"We sweat the small stuff, because it's not small stuff when patients are concerned," Bob Page said.

We sweat the small stuff, because nothing is small stuff when patients are concerned.

It's an exacting process that applies not only to patient safety, but to every aspect of operations because, "We question everything we're doing to see how we can do this better," said Tammy Peterman.

Getting the Questions Right

At KU Health System, the answer to every question is *Do the right thing for patients.* So asking the right questions is key, and everyone is engaged in that process from their own vantage point. From inner rings of higher management to outer rings of staff at the front lines, a circular organizational structure strengthens the network and the process. It engages everyone in participative, representative management.

HOW WE KNOW THAT

The Importance of Questioning What We Know

Back in 1998, we had nowhere to go but up. Improving our performance was not only *how* we survived, it was *why* we survived. We committed ourselves to learning how to put the patient first in everything we did, and we gained ground each time we got that right.

So we do "question it"—every day. For example, we weren't making progress in all areas of "zero harm." Patients were falling, getting pressure injuries...we had protocols in place, so why weren't we reaching our "zero" goals?

Chris Ruder, RN, chief operating officer, Kansas City Division, and a cadre of eight experts from leadership locked themselves in a room to dive deep into the issue—literally blocked themselves off from their regular workload to focus on zero harm exclusively for a week. Chris and his team explored this whole concept of *What do we think we know that we actually don't know...what haven't we gotten right?* What they found was we'd made a lot of assumptions about what we know. "We trained it" addresses only the people—not the process—so we had to look at that critically.

Focusing on ten of the most recent pressure injury cases, they noted that in 20 percent of them, providers placed different orders than were recommended by the wound team; an additional 20 percent showed nothing at all was done. The recommendations of the wound team experts were implemented as written 60 percent of the time, but it took two to five days for those orders to be entered by the provider.

Those delays were really significant. Not paying attention to the recommendations of the experts is a problem—and it also doesn't sound like our people. What Chris and his team discovered was *finding* those recommendations in the electronic medical record was really difficult. Staff was often unaware of what was being directed. So we had to make that easier and more actionable.

LEADERSHIP LESSON:

Staff was often unaware of what was being directed. So we had to make that easier and more actionable in the electronic medical record. This is the value of looking critically at a process—it underscores the trust our staff has earned, while fixing the problems that keep them from performing at their highest level.

Even though the things already on the zero-harm checklist were correct, asking more questions turned up six more things we should be doing—absolutely foundational steps.

Chris Ruder and his team explored every opportunity to hone in on solutions—like using our new SOS (Save Our Skin) Model to round with staff on patients with Stage 2 pressure injuries. By rounding in this manner, we were hardwiring the information into the work of the care provider right at the bedside.

Every way we can reinforce the information improves the process and enables staff to do it *right*.

When the goal is zero harm, the question is *What will it take to get to zero?*—not really, really close to zero. Even when the metrics are moving in the right direction, we have to keep asking questions until we reach zero, and then sustain zero harm.
—Tammy Peterman

The circular leadership structure works like a web or inter-connected network, not an old-school "rake" org chart where everything was controlled at the top and flowed down. This promotes the communication necessary to react quickly and effectively.

Bob Page believes, "In a word, it's *agility*. There's no stronger imperative for agility than a patient's needs, and no function in this health system that isn't related to patient care."

There's no stronger imperative for agility than a patient's needs, and no function in this health system that isn't related to patient care.

"Agility is a real asset to their success," Huron Consulting Group consultant Chris Drummond agreed. "KU Health System is more agile than other academic medical centers. Many AMCs require consensus for any decision. Representative management in decision-making is critical for agility. KU Health System's operating model allows it to make decisions with representative leadership instead of total consensus while achieving significant buy-in from the stakeholders—that's a huge advantage."[5]

Leadership at all levels provides a continuous flow of information in the representation process that supports agility. It means bench and bedside perspectives get shared all the way up to the executive board room. And those insights go hand-in-hand with the data, so organizational decisions get made more efficiently, functionally, and holistically.

Leadership at All Levels

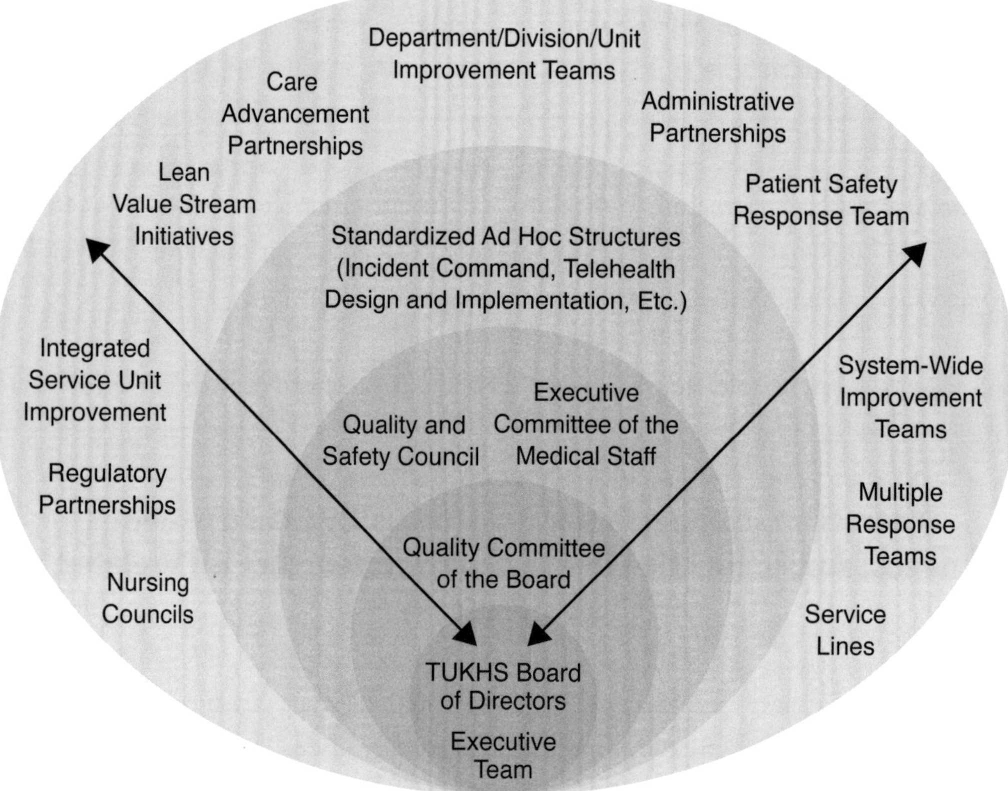

From the board to committees, partnerships, teams, and groups, the structure is designed to support organizational agility and leadership at all levels. Ongoing communication flows back and forth, but also around the circular network.

LEADERSHIP LESSON:

Representative management in decision-making is the key to agility. And it takes leadership at all levels to create an agile organization.

HOW WE KNOW THAT

The Data-Driven Answers to Quality of Care Questions

Why should you have to fly over Kansas to get heart care somewhere else when our results are comparable if not better than theirs, and we've got the data to prove it? Of course, we didn't always have that data. In fact, when I started here in '96, the only data we had showed how bad we were at keeping patients and staff happy. We committed to turning that completely around. Becoming a data-driven organization was key to that transformation.

In a world where Tammy Peterman's son-in-law managed a fast-food restaurant and knew the revenue and direct expense on an hourly basis, imagine a $2.5 billion business getting profitability data by service line and by diagnostic-related group every six months. That's not going to do much for your organizational agility!

But this isn't only about profit: Everything we do should be evidence-based and focused on our five stars, so we recalibrated. We did some things that were unprecedented in the industry at the time. I don't know any healthcare organization that was using patient satisfaction data as early as we were—in real-time based on patient discharge date—to analyze trends and patterns with unit-level specificity.

The point was, and continues to be, applying that information in ways that improve the patient experience. Today, our patient satisfaction and quality outcomes are among the best in the industry. But there's always more to know. We continue to build an infrastructure that supports data-mining, so when the numbers are red-flagging an issue, we've got the people and the process in place to address it.

In 2019, our focus on real-time data through Vizient identified an unfavorable trend. Our expected mortality, when compared with other comprehensive academic medical centers (CAMCs), suggested our outcomes were not as good as they had previously been, even though our actual mortality rate was very low. Something like that could impact how our performance is perceived in the local and national community, and how health insurance companies regard our care and their willingness to recommend us to their members. We had to address that disparity.

Analyzing our "expected" versus "actual" mortality rate presented us with a challenge. Although our rank in the top tier of AMCs nationwide had been steady for more than a decade, those great outcomes and low mortality rates were masking a subtle, underlying problem. The data supporting our quality of care was solid, so we had to dive deeper to get to the bottom of this. That's how we discovered we weren't consistently coding secondary diagnoses.

At an AMC, we see the sickest of sick patients. Their primary diagnosis is often severely complicated by secondary conditions that impact how acutely ill the patient is, but we weren't always documenting that level of patient acuity in the chart. Filling that gap required a process that more accurately captured the complexity of our patient mix. So we've proceeded the way we always do—collaborating and coaching with the *people* who do the work itself in order to fix the *process*.

The data always tells the story—or alerts us to the plot. Questioning our process turned up both problems and solutions. Now the needle is moving in the right direction on consistency with our expected and actual risk-adjusted mortality rate (RAMR), thanks to improvements in our coding process.

LEADERSHIP LESSON:

The data always tells the story—or alerts us to the plot.

When you're a data-driven organization, the quest is always to ask the right questions. Then you've got to believe what the data is telling you—especially the possibility that you're not asking all the right questions.
—Bob Page

LEADERSHIP LESSON:
When you're a data-driven organization, the quest is always to ask the right questions. Then you've got to believe what the data is telling you—especially the possibility that you're not asking all the right questions.

The Credibility Factor

There are complexities to generating data at an academic medical center, according to Associate Professor Keith Sale, MD, vice president and chief physician executive of ambulatory services.

"At an AMC, physicians are also trained as researchers and educators, so they're used to drawing on data or models derived from rigorous academic processes," Sale said. "The validation of the data and metrics we produce compared to various national benchmarks can be a challenge."

There are historical tensions embedded in this dynamic—the academic pursuit of the art and science of healing versus the agenda of a clinical business enterprise. Alignment of the two—each with its own distinct process and goals—isn't always in sync, or even possible.

Data must be reliable and relevant from the perspective of research and publication while also addressing the need for daily course corrections and direct applications in the clinical setting. Building trust and facilitating collaboration are crucial, so the data the health system creates will be reliable and relevant from an academic point of view, while enabling the necessary organizational agility.

LEADERSHIP LESSON:
The data the health system creates must be reliable and relevant from an academic point of view, while sustaining the necessary organizational agility.

With collaborative leadership at all levels and across disciplines, that burden is shared. Collecting, analyzing, and applying data to inform decisions and improve processes is a cross-functional team effort.

"Using data to inform medicine, care, decision-making, and improvement has been all about questioning our assumptions and beliefs over the years," Chief Culture Officer Terry Rusconi noted. "I can remember back when we believed ventilator-associated pneumonia was an expected complication for patients on vents. It was almost a given. Only when we questioned that foundational assumption did one of our teams come together to develop a ventilator-weaning protocol that virtually eliminated the problem for us. Questioning the accuracy of what we think we know is about continuous improvement."

It was that relentless pursuit that produced the IOS.

The Inpatient Operating System

The University of Kansas Health System's Inpatient Operating System, or IOS, didn't have a name yet when COO Chris Ruder and the nursing leadership team were developing it in 2019, but they did have a vision of what they wanted to do:

- Redefine the operating system within the inpatient unit with focus on two components
    - improvement system
    - management system
- Eliminate random, misunderstood variation
    - eradicate defects in process metrics
    - achieve and sustain zero-harm goal
- Develop a formula for sustained outcomes at or above goal
- Engage employees with high levels of ownership and satisfaction

They also had well-defined goals:

- Patient satisfaction consistently >90th percentile
- Zero harm (not just reduced harm, but zero harm)
- Employee engagement/satisfaction in the top decile
- LOS index <.85
- Direct cost index <1.0

And, best of all, the nursing leadership team had good reason to believe this was achievable. It just had to extrapolate what had been learned in Unit 62—the uber-achieving medical/telemetry "model cell"—across the entire KU Health System.

"Unit 62 was producing some incredible outcomes through their Lean work, and our goal was to replicate what they were doing unit by unit, and make it the norm system-wide," Chris Ruder explained.

How to Question It

Actually, what Unit 62 was doing began in 2014 when The University of Kansas Health System adopted "Lean" management principles. The Lean concept was to maximize uncompromised quality and value to the customer while eliminating waste in the process.[6] Originally developed by Toyota for auto production, Lean's efficient, continuous improvement process began to find its way into healthcare by the early 2000s. Its unique implementation at KU Health System is explored in detail in Chapter 6.

The IOS germinated in Lean and grew out of the answers to these questions relative to management and improvement:

- How can we question "it" the right way, and then do the right thing with the answer?
- How do we sustain that and share what we've learned system-wide?

How can we question "it" the right way, and then do the right thing with the answer—system-wide?

"It" was whatever needed improvement in process and patient safety. *Process* involved how to observe and, ultimately, use the data that was being produced by the IOS itself—tens of thousands of observations—to apply actionable knowledge to patient safety risks:

- CAUTI (catheter-associated urinary tract infection)
- CLABSI (central line-associated blood stream infection)
- Falls
- CDI/C. diff (clostridium difficile infection)
- HAPI (hospital-acquired pressure injury)

Discipline and Rigor (Not Quick and Easy)

"In every shift, seven days every week, the IOS imposes discipline and rigor to our process," Ruder explained. "Not just for individuals, but as unit teams, and even as executive management. There's not an easy button. You can't just quickly do it—that's not what it's about. It's about identifying the true problem, the target condition, and the steps toward sustained improvement."

We Go Slow to Go Fast

In healthcare, improvement is always the goal, but the focus is often lost when so many other things require attention. However promising an approach may be, improvement falls off because we move on to something else. We see it over and over again. Part of this work is to say we can't let something we worked so hard on, and improved, go in the other direction. We are locked into sustaining the gains that are made.

The gains sustained by Unit 62 for over five years don't need to be revisited again and again and again. We sustained what we did, kept it in place, then moved on to the next problem. We are trying to get that flywheel effect that builds and sustains this momentum system-wide. We can't do it if we keep jumping to put out the next fire or look at some shiny object.

The process can seem slow without immediate outcomes, but this is how we operate. We go slow to go fast. If you don't have the time to do it right, you're certainly not going to have the time to do it over again later. The IOS helps us figure out the right way to tackle it so we have to do it only once—that's efficient and effective. That may mean exercising the discipline to admit that no, we can't chase down another issue today because we're already focused on this problem. The IOS is about applying that kind of discipline and rigor toward our sustainable improvement goals.[7]
—Chris Ruder

LEADERSHIP LESSON:
We go slow to go fast. The IOS requires discipline and rigor to find the right way to tackle a problem so you have to do it only once, because if you don't have the time to do it right, you're certainly not going to have the time to do it over again later.

A Two-Part Plan for Continuous Improvement

Nurse Manager Miki Mahnke, RN, BSN, CMSRN, views IOS this way: "It's a two-part plan that provides tools and the leadership capacity to use them effectively. The Improvement System tools help ensure patient safety. The Management System helps me lead and develop my team so they know why they're using the tools and how to use them."

The Improvement System tools include:

- Zero-harm observation forms to identify risk factors and develop prevention strategies for each individual patient
- Team "huddles" scheduled four times across every shift to address specific aspects of care and risk prevention
- Quality "bundles" combining the essential, research-proven items and interventions to standardize zero-harm practices
- Small tests of change to trial PDSA (Plan/Do/Study/Act) and track the effectiveness of the improvement strategy
- "Kamishibai" boards to focus on observations of the work in progress versus a focus on the outcome

The Management System teaches leaders how to focus on achieving measurable, sustainable change by developing their teams' leadership and problem-solving skills.

The IOS provides the process infrastructure, tools, and management strategies for continuous improvement.

Integrating the improvement and management components of IOS created a reduction in patient-harm events that's been measurable, more predictable, and sustainable. It has provided the infrastructure, tools, and management strategies for continuous improvement. And over time, the IOS has significantly reduced—and in some areas actually eliminated—controllable risk factors in harm prevention.[8] (See Chapter 6: Improve It)

IOS: Proven Improvement

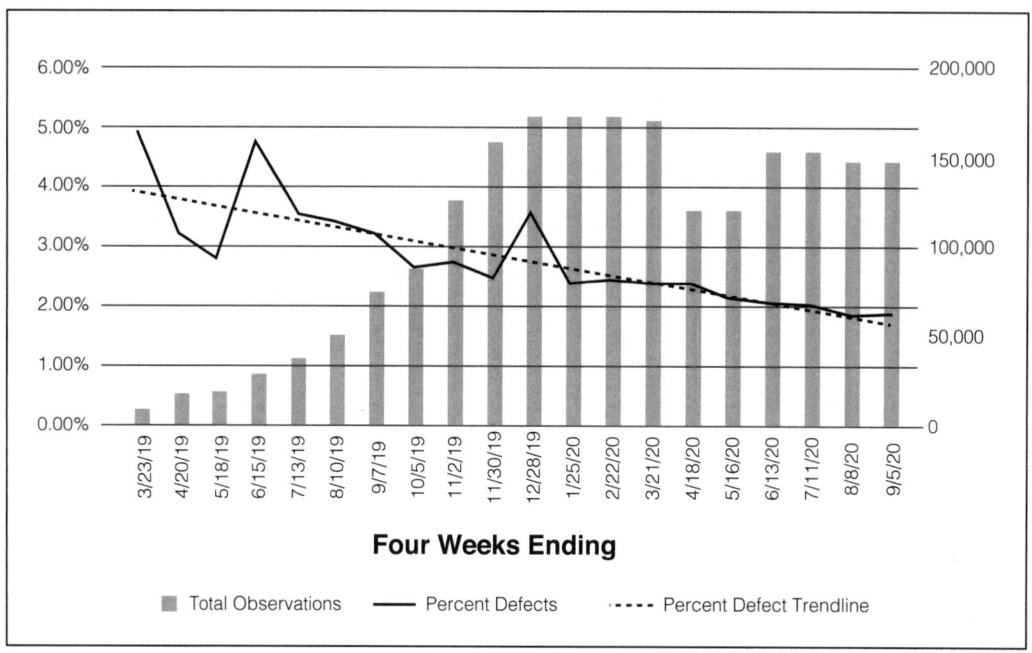

The discipline and focus compelled by IOS proved itself in its first year of implementation. With a 14-fold increase in observations and a more than 60 percent reduction in defect rates, harm events continue to trend toward the goal: zero.[9]

Lead Differently

Before IOS implementation, Mahnke's role was typical of nurse managers.

"My leadership philosophy used to be, *If I hire great people—the ones with good grades and good intentions—and be their biggest cheerleader, then good outcomes will follow*," she said.

Reports and problems reached Mahnke in her office, and regular meetings were scheduled to address concerns and stay abreast of what was happening on the floor.

LEADERSHIP LESSON:

Our Inpatient Operating System requires a new leadership style that's more engaged and instructional, not just directive. The focus is on developing the team.

But the IOS changed the role of leadership within the unit. In turn, Mahnke had to fundamentally change the way she interacted with employees.

"What I know now is I have to show staff how to observe and act—not just cheer them on louder," she explained. "I learned that I must be a teacher first and a cheerleader second. I'm more proactive, less reactive. IOS has provided me the tools to set clear, consistent expectations and a process to measure in real time if those expectations are being met."

The net result is patients receive more consistent care throughout the hospital.

"Prior to IOS, I was the manager on the unit racing around providing as much direct care as possible," Mahnke added. "IOS has given me confidence in my teams to provide the best, safest care."

With IOS, the leader's primary job is developing a team that has:

- the ability to recognize an issue in real time
- the skills to identify the root cause of the problem
- the knowledge of the target condition (the goal, where we want to be)
- the tools to improve it
- the discipline and rigor to sustain improvement (with IOS observation/questioning)

With IOS, individuals and teams are problem-solvers. They don't just react because their manager has alerted them to an issue. Individuals and the team are prepared to respond proactively with best practices.

Direct Data Dosing

Another IOS impact changed the manager's relationship to the data. In the past, managers received data monthly or quarterly.

Post-IOS implementation, Mahnke said, "I receive data twice daily to measure how the team is performing in harm-reduction categories. This real-time data promotes quicker intervention, and allows us to put a stop in place to prevent patient harm."[10]

> IOS also allows me to have a closer relationship with patient satisfaction. Twice daily, bedside leaders send me communication about customer service opportunities—what service recovery was provided and the response. We've achieved sustainable, predictable high patient satisfaction scores with the daily focus on rounding with intent on every patient two times every day.
> —Miki Mahnke

The IOS generates real-time data that translates to actionable knowledge informing management about both patients and staff. Nurse managers regularly work side by side with staff to provide coaching and encouragement, and to keep questioning "it" at eye-contact level.

The goal has been to continuously identify opportunities for improvement, then test them through actionable steps that result in new and better practices that are sustainable.

For example, when it became apparent through IOS observations that longer tubing was a problem for patients with in-dwelling urinary catheters, a team immediately went to the simulation lab to figure out different ways to solve for this. Tubing should allow uninterrupted, free-flow drainage to avoid infection, but the product length often made that impractical.

"We don't want to ask staff to do something that's not possible with the current products we have," Ruder explained, adding that ideas are developed and implemented using small tests of change. Nurses devised various approaches to position and secure the tubing.

Even using a pillowcase to help guide the tube's movement as the patient shifted in bed proved surprisingly effective.

"Our internal innovations team continues to work on its own device or product that might have potential here," Ruder added.

The entire process is focused on addressing the issues *in situ*—localized to the actual place with the people who are experiencing them.

"Assumptions and beliefs get reality-checked by data and human connection—actionable knowledge and actual names," said Chris Ruder. "The goal is to get to the root cause in real time."

Assumptions and beliefs get reality-checked by data and human connection—actionable knowledge and actual names. The goal is to get to the root cause in real time.

"IOS is a completely different approach," Tammy Peterman said. "We don't tell people not to have meetings, but if they're doing this right, leadership is spending a lot more time where the work is done. Our future state is not to be reliant on retrospective reports or data, but to have real-time knowledge and the ability to apply it."

LEADERSHIP LESSON:

To find a sustainable solution, the root cause of problems must be identified in real time, not from a data review after the fact. What we're learning through IOS work is how to develop employees who have the skills to do exactly that—solve problems on the spot or, even better, prevent problems from occurring.

Data becomes information, and information becomes actionable knowledge.

"On Unit 62, the team wasn't waiting for Tori Butler, RN (former nurse manager of Unit 62), to point out the problem; the team could do that itself," Chris Ruder explained. "This isn't a skillset you just turn on; you have to build it. Building that takes some time. Education, training, and practice of our principles. That's IOS. We are in practice every day, and we're getting better...more competent. We believe that practice is critical, and that requires discipline and rigor."[11]

Competency Builds Capacity

To build competency is to build capacity. Consistent with leadership at all levels, with IOS, the work of improvement isn't trickle-down; it's circular and self-educating.

"We share what we learn a lot of different ways from many sources," said Quality & Safety Director Amanda Gartner. "We learn from the defects that are uncovered by IOS. We learn every single day about work flow, supply issues, and what the patient needs—from being on the front line with staff and as staff."[12]

LEADERSHIP LESSON:

To build competency is to build capacity.

Everyone is climbing the learning curve from various angles, contributing to the data, and sharing knowledge. One of the most immediate, accessible mechanisms for that is "the huddle."

Huddle Up

Huddles aren't uncommon in healthcare, but the IOS calls for even more of them to optimize communication—the kind that keeps the unit informed on all fronts and connects staff going off or on shift. Each huddle has a specific focus and is facilitated to ensure that everyone participates in the agenda:

- **Command Center** huddles happen before every shift to update and alert staff on patients and specific risk factors that can be preemptively avoided.

- **Interdisciplinary** huddles happen during every shift; representatives from medical practice, nursing, OT/PT, speech therapy, dietary, pharmacy, chaplaincy, social work, and case management discuss and plan a cohesive approach to addressing unique issues for each patient.
- **Daily Status Report** huddles at 10:30 a.m. engage the unit coordinator or charge nurse and the nursing manager on:
    - Patient safety concerns that were raised during rounds
    - Any defects that were reported and related coaching that was provided
    - Team-building and professional development goals
    - Patient- and family-stated concerns or problems and the plans to resolve them
    - Any new medical device or a trial
    - Whatever else needs to be discussed
- **MDI (Measuring Daily Improvement)** is the huddle for the nursing team to discuss progress on improvements—how are we doing on this test of change? Were there any near misses, any defects…what was learned? Measuring quality and improvement progress is the focus.

From huddles come innovations. Everyone is engaged in the conversation—not just listening to others talk. When some of the nurses were struggling with pressure sore preventions, Mahnke said huddles provided a solution.

"We decided to trial 'turn teams' to help us with safe patient handling," she said. "So instead of a nurse turning her four patients every two hours all by herself, we tried two nurses teaming up and turning the patients together. This helped us with body mechanics while it strengthened our team approach. And all of that helps with patient safety and staff burnout."

A strategy like turning teams could be trialed for a week and adapted if the practice is helpful. *How* helpful it is will show up in the observation data. Even the huddles present ripe opportunities for observation. During a Command Center huddle with the nurses on the unit, there are often members of management and even executive leadership joining in to observe and engage. The synergy influences the delivery of care that day, and the holistic approach to administration of the health system on the broad scale.

The Inpatient Operating System is an unprecedented approach to joining the fluidity of innovation to a structured approach for continuous improvement.

"I remember when Chris Ruder brought all the nurse managers together and told us we would build this process together," Mahnke reflected. "Every single one of us had a big part to play. It's always about tying this process back to the patient—keeping it real and personal. When someone comes in for a transplant and leaves with a UTI—that's on us. We have to own that so we can learn and do better. IOS is about owning it, learning from it, and doing better."

It all comes back to focusing on the patient and the spirit of constant improvement, according to Kansas City Division CNO Rachel Pepper, DNP.

"I think much of our innovation and improvement stems from engaging our people as a team and giving them the power to question our processes every day," Pepper said. "Innovation, in the spirit of improving the safety of our patients, is constantly at play. This important work has been a natural complement to our culture."

CHAPTER SIX

Improve It

Continuous improvement is better than delayed perfection.
—Mark Twain

It's not a secret room, but there are no directional signs to it. Its out-of-the-way location in the corner of a lower-level parking garage is intentional. This is the *Obeya* room at KU Health System. It is "command central" where representatives of executive leadership, management, and staff leave their titles at the door and join in a collaborative continuous improvement process that's been going on, in one form or another, for over 20 years.

"We didn't know closeting ourselves away was a 'Lean' concept when we tried it the first time," admitted Tammy Peterman, explaining that in 2001, several members of the leadership team locked themselves in a room and didn't go back to their offices or work stations until they came up with a viable methodology to improve patient medical records. At that time, it was a blended system of paper and electronic records, often making it hard to navigate and find information quickly.

"Back then, it was the 'No more whining, no more complaining, no more money, no more people—now let's come together and work this out' room," she laughed.

Today, it's the Obeya Room—ground zero for the health system's Lean data visualization, information-sharing, problem-solving, and improvement-planning.

Back then, it was the "No more whining, no more complaining, no more money, no more people—now let's come together and work this out" room.

A Humble but Big Bang

The evolution of continuous improvement that would eventually produce the rigorous Inpatient Operating System (IOS) at The University of Kansas Health System in 2019 (see Chapter 5) had its big bang back in 1998 when it was freed up to function autonomously.

"Frankly, we had nowhere to go but up when we split off from the state system," Bob Page pointed out. "We had the lowest patient satisfaction ranking in the country at that time—in the 5th percentile—but as a newly independent hospital, we were finally in a position to do something about that."

To that end, initiatives focused on improving performance on the "big dot" measures were implemented, but the most important factor in the unparalleled transformation of TUKHS was the culture itself. By 2007, the organization had reached the 90th percentile for patient satisfaction, and it has held rank as a top performing hospital ever since.[1]

Big Dot Performance Improvements

The work to improve "big dot" performance involved both large and small process improvements as hospital leaders described system-wide change efforts [in 2001]. Hand-offs between caregivers, especially at nursing shift changes, now required safety huddles to discuss patients. Teams of two nurses carried out additional safety checks. Rapid response teams focused on patients whose condition had deteriorated. An acute stroke response team was formed to deliver critical care specialists to a patient's bedside within five minutes.

Determining co-morbidities and severity of illness at admission helped lead the hospital to implement standardized coding systems that contributed to better patient tracking.

> [Former CEO] Irene Thompson also supported an initiative proposed by the medical staff to conduct a mortality review for each hospital death in an effort to identify service, system, or other changes that might avert the same outcome for future cases. Mortality scores improved even as the hospital's case mix index (a measure of patient diversity, clinical complexity, and resource needs) grew more complex by an average of 1.8 percent a year.[2]
> —Arthur Daemmrich, PhD

Both Page and Peterman credit the culture for the organic nature of continuous improvement at KU Health System. While variable improvement methodologies have been tried to good effect, the constant has been the people applying them.

"Continuous improvement is hardwired into our culture—it doesn't just come from whatever new method is trending," Page said. "It comes from within the people who are functioning optimally if leadership is doing its job."

LEADERSHIP LESSON:

Continuous improvement is hardwired into our culture—it doesn't come externally from whatever new method is trending. It comes from within the people who are functioning optimally if leadership is doing its job.

Try, Trying, Tried

Historically, improvement methodologies in healthcare have been adopted from industry. Engineer W. Edwards Deming's Plan, Do, Study, Act inspired the Hospital Corporation of America (HCA)'s FOCUS-PDCA (Plan, Do, Check, Act), an improvement process that was in place at KUH and probably every other hospital in the '90s. The Institute for Healthcare Improvement (IHI) introduced its adaptation, the Rapid Cycle Improvement Model, during this time as well.[3] As other promising methods mustered in from '98 to

'08, KU Hospital tried and applied them, optimizing the best of each and enhancing it in context to its culture.

- **FOCUS-PDCA**, mid '90s
  Find a process; Organize a team; Clarify current knowledge; Understand variability and capability; Select a plan for continuous improvement—to Plan, Do, Check, Act with controlled tests measuring discrete results that drive further improvements.

- **IHI Rapid Cycle**, 1999
  Improvement Model (using PDCA)
  Apply three questions to the PDCA cycle: What are we trying to accomplish? How will we know that a change is an improvement? What change can we make that will result in improvement?

- **GM PICOS**, 2001
  From General Motors, a Program for the Improvement and Cost Optimization of Suppliers (PICOS) that uses Lean approaches to facilitate supplier cost reductions.

- **Failure Mode and Effects Analysis (FMEA)**
  A systematic method of identifying and preventing product and process problems before they occur. It had been used in many industries to prevent bad things from happening.

- **100,000 Lives Campaign**, 2004
  Then-IHI president and CEO Don Berwick, MD, challenged the healthcare industry to save 100,000 lives in 18 months with six specific interventions: deploy rapid response teams; deliver reliable, evidence-based care for acute myocardial-infarction; prevent adverse drug events; prevent central line infections; prevent surgical site infections; prevent ventilator-associated pneumonia. In 2006, this was expanded to focus on reducing incidents of patient harm by five million.

"We would work to understand the essential elements of an approach, customize it to best work within the organization, and then add it to enhance the methods already in place," Terry Rusconi, who was then director of organizational development, explained. "Other than FOCUS-PDCA, they're still all a differentiated part of the performance improvement DNA of this health system. Improvement is really the essence of our mantra: *We're proud but never satisfied.*"

Show Me the Cost Savings

As thin as the margin was, profitability wasn't specifically targeted for improvement, but fiscal management was. All the rigor around service, quality, and people would now be applied to sustainability.

In 2012, the Huron Consulting Group was engaged to enhance productivity, reduce expenses, and improve operational performance. Eight primary areas were targeted: Clinical Operations, Human Resources, Clinical Documentation, Managed Care, Non-Labor, Physician, Labor, and Facility Life. The goal was to continue delivering superior care but at significantly lower costs—without layoffs. KU Hospital then-CFO Bill Marting developed the E5 as its delivery model.

The E5 Improvement Model

Every day, The University of Kansas Hospital will lead the nation through its primary focus on

Excellence in patient care, enabled by

Efficiency in operations,

Expense management supportive of future growth and investment, and

Execution of best practices second to none in speed and thoroughness of implementation

"One of the first things we did was start sharing financial information with physicians," Page recalled. "Physicians needed to know if Medicare was going to pay for only five days of a patient's seven-day stay, not to encourage an unsafe discharge at day five, but to let them help us figure out where efficiency could be improved to safely progress the patient through the care process."

It was a constant education. Tammy Peterman described the impact, "We knew we had to manage differently. For example, if we could reduce the length of stay but still get people what they need when they need it, that's better for the patient. It's also better for the organization, and it gets the next patient in the door in a more expedited fashion."

We began to see incremental improvement. By fiscal year 2018, "We had a .5-day reduction in length of stay," Peterman pointed out. "The reduction in stay might not seem like a lot, but it's a tremendous amount, resulting in an additional available 55 beds per day without any expansion of the physical space."

In fact, one month during that fiscal year, the lowest-ever length of stay was documented.[4]

"That isn't because we reduced the amount of care; it's because we delivered care with greater efficiency and less wait time," clarified Peterman. "It's better for the patient to have a shorter length of stay."

> As a society, we have created a health system that is driven around what's best for the clinician and not what's best for the patient. We have not designed our systems around the patient; we've designed them around the physicians, the nurses, and everybody else. We're now being asked to provide the same level—if not higher level—of care for less money. We can't get there, in my opinion, doing it the way we've always done it. So, I think this is a challenge to fundamentally redesign how we manage and operate, and it starts from the patient's perspective, not from the doctor's, or nurse's, or executive's perspective.[5]
>
> —Bob Page

In collaboration, KU Health System and Huron identified more than 120 initiatives to improve resource utilization and expense reduction. Comprehensive staffing matrices, shift management tools, and detailed work flow analyses improved performance while keeping the organization's commitment to no layoffs. All told, more than $60 million of annually recurring benefit was generated against a target of $48 million. The engagement also provided an additional one-time cost-savings benefit of $9 million due to reduction in inventory levels as well as modifying facility life.[6] Equally important, E5 also created a wide range of standardized practices to sustain these improvements.

Equally important, E5 also created a wide range of standardized practices to sustain these improvements.

The E5 methodology marked the beginning of increasingly tailored improvement strategies for The University of Kansas Health System.

- **E5**, 2013 – 2017
  From Huron Consulting Group, E5 focused Every day on Efficiency in operations, Execution of best practices, Excellence in patient care, and Expense management supportive of future growth and investments.

- **Lean**, 2014
  From Toyota, a continuous improvement process that eliminates waste without sacrificing quality.

- **IOS**, 2019
  TUKHS in-house-generated Inpatient Operating System that incorporates the lessons of transformation and expands on Lean with KU Health System's uniquely differentiated application.

HOW WE KNOW THAT

From the 5th to the 95th Percentile: The Secret to Vast Improvement

When I came to KU Hospital in 1996 as the vice president of organizational improvement (a department of one), there were challenges on every front. I wasn't sure what to take on first, so I decided to look at performance improvement by comparing our performance to other organizations based on data from the University HealthSystem Consortium.

I got a lot of pushback from doctors telling me, "That data is not accurate. You can't survey and compare us with Johns Hopkins, because we are different." Okay, to whom can I compare us? How about to other people here? The answer was, "No, you can't do that; physicians are too different." So finally, I had a huge realization: *How about I compare you to you?* But I had to do that as an ally, not an enemy. Improvement doesn't work unless everyone is engaged toward the goal.

Gradually, I built spreadsheets on different types of surgery, tracking *wheels in—cut time, close time—wheels out, white space, and the next case.* Relationships between physicians and process got clearer. As the data grew, I could see ways to improve processes and make efficiency gains, but it was difficult to use the information to drive changes. It wasn't until we split off from the university in '98 that this hospital could engage in a clinical agenda of viable improvement.

It wasn't just a slogan in an advertisement or annual report; it was the secret sauce that made everything we were doing work because it was always, without question, the right thing to do.

The most important thing we did to orient this institution toward improvement was engage everyone in the process. We leveraged their expertise into a process of putting the patient first in every decision we made as a board, as executives, and as staff. For us, it wasn't just a slogan in an advertisement or annual report; it was the secret sauce that made everything we were doing work because it was always, without question, the right thing to do. For staff, knowing leadership had their back increased confidence and trust. Doing the right thing transformed our culture and created our business model.

From our Press Ganey low point at the 5th percentile for patient satisfaction in 1997, to a sustained position in the top 20 percent of hospitals nationwide since 2006, and the top 10 percent of hospitals today,[7] our continuous improvement culture has evolved proactively. Today, we are developing and implementing IOS, a continuous improvement model that's unprecedented anywhere else in the industry. And we're doing it the same way we've always done it—consistent with the culture of this health system. —Bob Page

Headed in the Right Direction with Patient Satisfaction

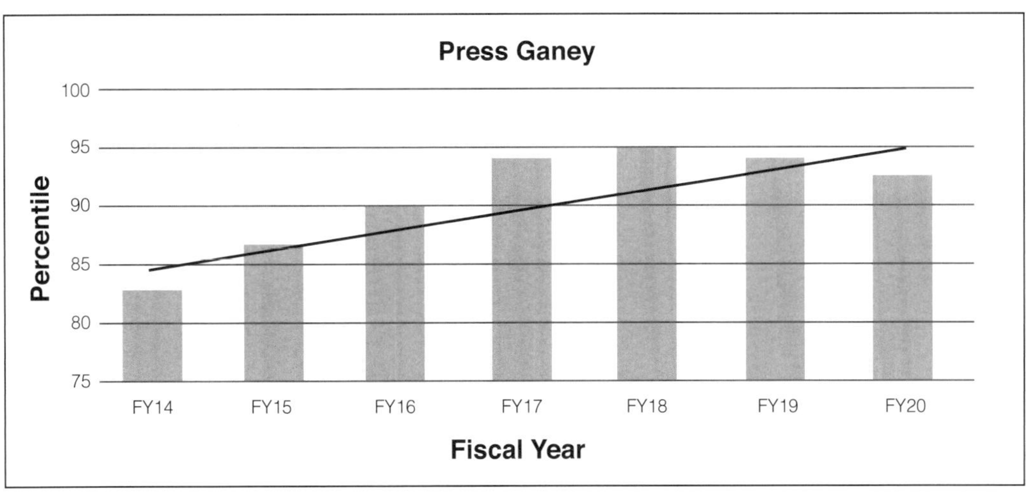

LEADERSHIP LESSON:

The most important thing we did to orient this institution toward improvement was engage everyone in the process. We leveraged their expertise into a process of putting the patient first in every decision we made as a board, as executives, and as staff.

A Lean Machine

Originally developed by Toyota in the 1950s to increase manufacturing productivity, the Lean management method looks at ways to enhance systems by eliminating defects and waste in processes. Philosophically, Lean seeks to align the workforce to a common goal of excellence in delivering value to the customer.[8]

"Lean management is a way of thinking—not just a set of tools or a checklist. It's an approach that fits our culture," Tammy Peterman explained.

Thanks to a patient-first culture and their Five-Star Guiding Formula (see Chapter 2), "We had already transformed this hospital into a nationally ranked health system, so for us, Lean wasn't the vehicle for that," Peterman said. "But Lean provided infrastructure as a continuous improvement model."

Their anticipatory approach was distinct because, as Lean expert and national healthcare consultant Mike Rona pointed out, "Usually, companies turn to Lean to fix a problem or even save the ship. At KU Health System, Lean was proactively implemented to build on the transformation that had already been achieved. It's part of their 'never rest on your laurels' belief system."

LEADERSHIP LESSON:

Customizing Lean to meet our needs required proactively (not reactively) applying its principles to fit our continuous improvement culture. We wanted to develop the organizational capacity and capability to plan ahead in light of pressures to do more with less that everyone was facing in the healthcare industry.

Lean in Every Value Stream

Although 2014 was a banner year for KU Health System—having received the largest research grant in the hospital's history and being ranked in the top 50 in all twelve data-driven specialties by *U.S. News & World Report*—Peterman and Page knew the pressures on healthcare organizations would continue to increase, especially from external regulatory agencies and governmental payers. They wanted to develop the organizational capacity and capability to preemptively tackle those challenges.

After a visit to Seattle's Virginia Mason Hospital where Lean had turned the tides with then-president/CEO Mike Rona's help, "We came back knowing we needed to do this," Page said. "And people got on board. Having a strong and conducive culture already in place helped us get over the resistance-to-change hurdles."

People got on board. Having a strong and conducive culture already in place helped us get over the resistance-to-change hurdles.

> The problem is if everything has to be done or led by two people, you don't have much leverage. You need to have the entire leadership leading this way. If you have 100-200 people leading this way, you can totally galvanize and leverage thousands of workers.
> —Mike Rona

Building on a foundation of success, the Lean journey at KU Health System began in earnest in 2014.

"It was akin to Michael Jordan hiring a personal trainer after an MVP season," acknowledged KU Hospital Authority Board Chairman Greg Graves. Dr. David Wild, an anesthesiologist on staff, was invited to take on an executive leadership role as vice president of Lean promotion.

Atypical of how most AMCs work, the organization was purposeful in looking for a leader from inside the organization who had a passion for wanting to make things better and who could become a Lean expert. Dr. Wild demonstrated all of that in the very first Lean Leadership sessions.

First order of business: Prioritize the units or processes in most need of Lean, a.k.a. *value streams*. The Lean approach begins at the end of the value stream and progresses toward the beginning.[9] Each value stream involves many departments, so much coordinated effort would be required to accomplish strategic objectives.

As Wild saw it, "The goal was to improve efficiency in all 14 value streams from perioperative services to inpatient care to HR, revenue cycle, supply chain, pharmacy, cancer care, and more. We cover the gamut of both patient care in clinical services and what would previously have been referred to as support or business services."

There would be some degree of savings, but Wild emphasized, "We never ask a team to identify a cost-reduction measure. We check it and follow it on the back end, but that's not the goal of the work."

> From the very beginning, Lean wasn't delegated. No manager is working from a slide-deck from HR, but from firsthand, frontline engagement in Kaizen and Gemba events. Executive leaders were at the first Kaizen event, and they've team-led Kaizen workshops. They are present at every Lean report-out given on Friday mornings. I can't overstate the importance of this—we were Lean at all levels. This is how Lean became thoroughly acculturated at this health system, not just a fad.
> —David Wild

Wild prioritized the value streams and developed the launch plan for weeklong rapid performance improvement workshops called *Kaizen* (a Japanese term meaning *change for the better*) events. In each value stream unit/department, a multi-disciplinary team—including those from the targeted area as well as others with an outsider perspective—would receive training on the Lean improvement model and tools. An executive-level leader or sponsor would present the problem, then set the group loose to rapidly try as many ideas as possible that week. The objective was to improve the process and identify the measures by which the goal was achieved.

Then the idea was put to the test, starting in the operating room.

HOW WE KNOW THAT

Making Better Problem-Solvers and Decision-Makers

The OR world is big, busy, and complex. On many days, we could have well over 100 people here for surgery. In 2014, that number was growing quickly, but we weren't in a position to expand our operating rooms. We had to find a way to do more cases safely in the given space, and that's how our first Lean conversations got started.

To address the OR challenge, we prioritized perioperative services—that's where we formally started our Lean journey. Our goal was to reduce wait times; improve the overall experience for patients; and make the system work better for patients, surgeons, anesthesiologists, and staff.

We identified our multidisciplinary team—25 of us—and we all went through Lean management training, including Dr. Delcore, chair of surgery; Bob; and me. Our first Kaizen event began at 5:15 a.m. upon patients' arrival. With their permission, each of us tracked one individual through his or her entire experience. From admitting all the way into the operating room and then afterward to the PACU (post-anesthesia care unit), we learned a lot.

Doing this Lean "Gemba" walk is about observing the patterns of how staff thinks and acts in the workplace so we can explore efficiencies together. Even participating surgeons who'd practiced here for 30 years admitted they were surprised by what they learned about this hospital by walking in a patient's shoes.

We discovered a great deal of duplication. Patients have to answer a list of questions in one place, then we'd ask the same questions—plus or minus a couple—at the next stop. We already knew that was an issue, but experiencing that alongside a patient really had impact. We observed a lot of wait time—both for patients and providers. Whether for documents to be signed or for the next physician to arrive, there was too much "hurry-up and wait" for all parties involved. It was a waste of time for patients and for our staff and physicians.

Linking various systems and processes could optimize the care being provided and make the experience better for patients and the care team. Kaizen events put management right there with the people who do this every day where it is happening—that's the beauty of Gemba. Being present in the workplace as the work was being done gave us insight into how to trouble-shoot and problem-solve together. From all these different perspectives, everyone brings his or her own expertise to find those opportunities for streamlining.

They weren't doing it in the most efficient way, because we hadn't given them an efficient system to work in.

Considering the challenges, I was amazed by what was happening in our hospital. Even in perioperative services, a system filled with barriers, great work was taking place. Day in and day out, staff would develop a work-around to provide the very best experience possible for patients and families. They weren't doing it in the most efficient way, because we hadn't given them an efficient system to work in. Kaizen helped with that. We identified many small, incremental steps to eliminate wasted time and effort. And Lean-thinking became the approach staff uses to address challenges even now. It's made all of us better problem-solvers and decision-makers.
—Tammy Peterman

The Model Cell

The staff of Unit 62 huddles at the beginning of every shift. Side chatter stills as the business at hand is swiftly addressed: the patient who is a fall risk…an update from morning rounds…questions about a new piece of equipment…head-counting who's attending the training workshop later that week.

Such huddles aren't uncommon on other units, but Tori Butler, RN, noted that as the model cell testing ground for all Lean process improvement for inpatient acute care, Unit 62 is different.

"But that's not the point," asserted Butler, who was Unit 62 nurse manager when the Medical Telemetry Unit 62 became the model cell. "The point is we *all* want to be different in the same way."

That "way" has been to reach unprecedented levels of achievement across numerous fronts, including 1,000 days without a blemish to the unit's zero-harm record (for catheter-associated urinary tract infections or CAUTI) and consistent patient satisfaction rankings above the 95th percentile.[10]

Unit 62: Reducing Harm

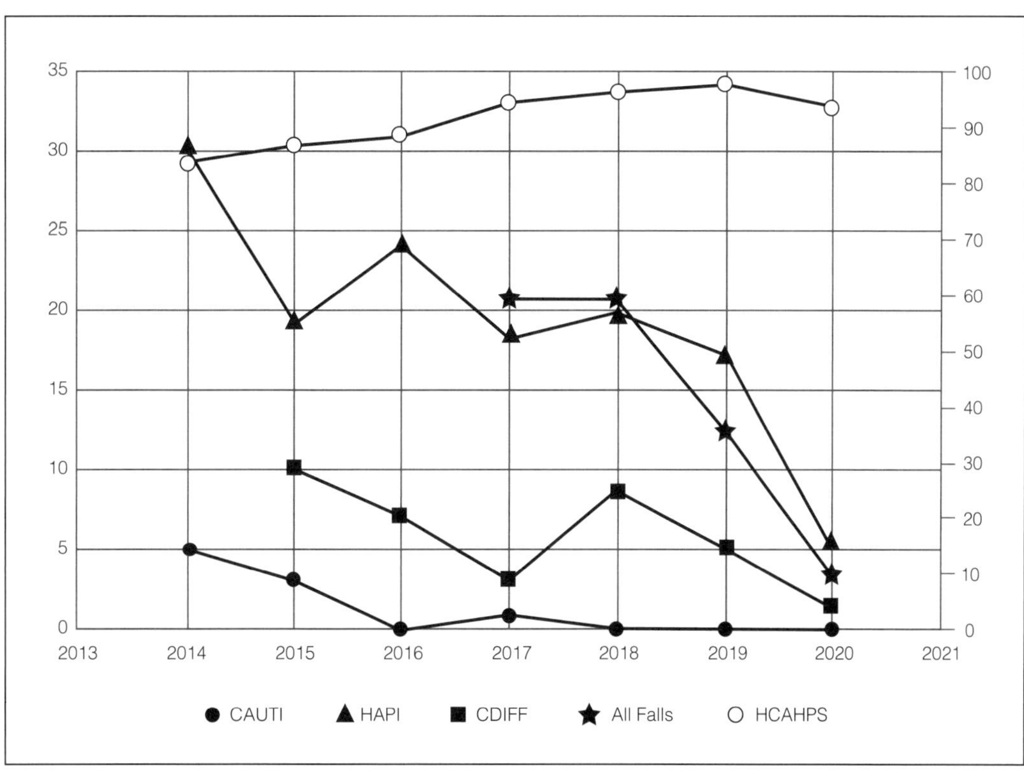

Unit 62 Achievements

Starting in 2014, there was a week-long Kaizen workshop every six to eight weeks all the way through 2016. Problems identified were solved, new ideas evolved, collaboration engaged, and leadership empowered from those workshops.

"It was a bit intense," Butler admitted. "We've gotten used to a rapid rate of change on this unit."

Unit 62's Medical Director Matt Jones, DO, added, "This is a team that wants to be pushed."

For each improvement or idea, rigorous monitoring was maintained for at least 90 days. During that period, Butler, Jones, and team would work through barriers to ensure they were doing the right work for both the patient and the team while also achieving the goals. Close data-tracking indicated what trended favorably and if the change was impactful.

"From there, it was decided if we would adopt the new practice into our standard of care," Butler explained. "We met all of our goals within the first year. Over six years later, we are sustaining those goals."

Measuring Up and Reporting Out

Unit 62 data-tracking was done on a daily basis.

"We learned how to look at processes through the patient's eyes and continually work to remove waste in the system, to avoid work-arounds, and to improve the current state," Butler said.

Progress and value stream metrics were reported weekly to Chris Ruder, RN. And every one to three weeks, that progress was reported out to the full executive leadership team that was focused not only on the big picture, but on the small details that could optimize the role of each staff member.

"We call that operating at the top of your licensure," said David Wild, MD.

Large or small, every opportunity to improve was engaged.

"That could mean an alcohol pad needed at the bedside is there when you need it so you can most effectively do your work," Wild explained. "You don't have to walk all over the place looking for an alcohol pad while making the patient wait. We will help you find ways to get those things you need where you need them."

What Comes After 62

What's been learned on Unit 62 gets shared across other units and departments. "It all crosses," Matt Jones said.

Numerous innovations have been implemented system-wide including:

- **Safety rounds with the four Ps** (potty, pain, positioning, and personal items) that emphasize verbalizing patient needs intentionally and proactively
- **Teach-back methodology** that educates and engages patients when staff is delivering medications
- **Pre-set discharge date and time** expectations to decrease delays, specifically around patient and family rides
- **Best rounding practices** with docs as the new standard of care for internal medicine physicians

At The University of Kansas Health System, our Lean work is shared and expanded through a tier system; each tier "feeds" the next tier. The most detailed work happens at Tier 3, the MDI (Managing Daily Improvements) that's done at the unit level with the frontline team every single shift. The focus is on improvements in the areas of quality, service, growth, people, and sustainability. In each area, we have an outcome metric (lag metric) and a process metric (lead metric). The team works through process improvement and monitors the progress here. The barriers or "defects" are identified on a Pareto chart to help us identify the next areas of focus for PDCA that will help impact the outcome metric.

This process engages the frontline team in continual daily improvement. The team feels empowered by the changes and takes ownership to continually build on these gains.

Tier 2 is focused on those value stream metrics (consistent identified metrics) plus the new implementation targets and run charts. The individual who oversees the value stream is the process owner. He or she keeps the work moving, eliminates barriers, surfaces concerns as they arise, and reports details of the work and weekly updates in progress to the executive-level sponsor.

The sponsor presents this information in broad terms to Tier 1, the entire executive team, for up to ten minutes. Tier 1 executives have another five to eight minutes to ask questions.
—Tori Butler and Matt Jones

Differentiating Lean

What differentiates Lean the most at KU Health System is the emphasis on proactivity and positivity. Thinking "Lean" in advance not only avoids anticipatable problems, it accelerates progress. Downtime that would be spent trouble-shooting, working-around, and retraining is available for innovation and improvement. It's the difference between fire prevention and firefighting.

"It's also about engaging our frontline staff differently," said Vice President of Cancer Services Jeff Wright. "It builds on our culture of engaging our frontline staff to improve systems supporting patient care and service."

At the Richard and Annette Bloch Cancer Care Pavilion, input from nurses on the size of the individualized treatment rooms led to a better design with appropriate space for patients and caregivers.

"Even when we designed Cambridge Tower A, we used Lean to plan the urgent and emergent pathways to optimize our rapid response teams," said Adam Meier, MSN, RN, chair of the Nursing Operations Advisory Council at TUKHS.

LEADERSHIP LESSON:

Thinking ahead with Lean is the difference between fire prevention and firefighting. It views problems as the raw materials from which improvements are made.

Thinking ahead with Lean means problems are seen as the raw materials from which improvements are made, and many innovations can be "pre-improved." Terry Rusconi put it this way, "Lean gave our culture-path a systems-path to follow."

LEADERSHIP LESSON:

Lean gave our culture-path a systems-path to follow...

- If something is needed to improve care, there's a mechanism in place to get it.
- If there's a barrier to providing the best care, there are steps in place to report it and resolve it.
- If someone has an idea that could create a better patient experience, there's a whole team ready to try it.

Getting Everyone in the Same Room

As the lessons learned on Unit 62 were shared, Colette Lasack's department was one of the early adopters.

Even in the billing process, "We're here to take care of patients," said Lasack, VP of revenue cycle. "They get the best care on the planet here, and we don't want to undo that a week later with a big, unexpected bill in the mail. We want the explanation of benefits from their insurance company to assure them their claim was processed and paid correctly. Then we've delivered the financial care we want to provide."

Patients get the best care on the planet here, and we don't want to undo that a week later with a big, unexpected bill in the mail.

During their first Kaizen event, they formulated a three-year strategy to simplify the billing and payment process with a goal of getting it right for each patient the first time, and every time. And since then, virtually everything in the revenue cycle gets a Lean vetting. To date, Lasack's department has done over 20 Kaizen events.

"We did one on authorization denials and found a disconnect between case management nurses and what was going out on the actual claim to the insurance company," Lasack said.

The insurance company's case management viewed three days of a five-day stay as outpatient/observation. According to Lasack, "Our system didn't have a good way for that to be communicated to us in billing."

Getting all the right people in the room was key.

"By bringing the clinical perspective and the denials follow-up teams together, we were able to clearly identify what standardized communication and work needed to happen—who needed to do what, where, and when," Lasack explained. "Together, we created consistent algorithms and standardized the language throughout the work streams.

"Administratively, everything is about three things—people, process, and technology," she added. "Those three things have to be aligned to get it right for the patient the first time and every time."[11]

LEADERSHIP LESSON:

Administratively, everything is about three things—people, process, and technology. Those three things have to be aligned to get it right for the patient the first time and every time.

Lean Leadership

We enhanced aspects of our nurse navigator program to ask, *Where is the waste?* We focused on referrals. Seems easy—they can come via email, fax, or a self-referral, and each type is handled quite differently. We analyzed all three types with the workshop team in the department. We quickly recognized a large amount of overprocessing and defects. We focused on balancing the workflow between the intake staff members as well as decreasing time wasted on hunting for specific clinical answers. We also evaluated the duplication that was occurring between team members who were maintaining multiple logs in various places.

With the changes that were implemented, we improved the referral cycle time by 40 percent. This allowed staff to ensure communications were clear and decisions were accurate, versus rushing through the work to answer the next call.

That was my first Lean workshop in the team leadership role. Our team included a nurse navigator and intake coordinator who understood the current process. However, everyone else involved—IT, revenue cycle, patient access, pre-registration—didn't directly know the process, or each other for that matter. Even so, there was a wonderful feeling of camaraderie as all titles stayed at the door—everyone collaborated as a peer. By Day 5, we had identified quite a bit of heavy lifting that needed to be done within the next 30 days.

Team member Shelonta McAfee, an intake coordinator who hadn't had a formal leadership role yet, actually volunteered to take on one of the biggest challenges, which included a brand-new phone referral standard work process. To me, this was such an excellent example of our culture. Shelonta volunteered to take this item because she felt secure and knew she would be supported along the way.

> That was such an important takeaway for me. We need to make changes to improve our process, and Lean helps with that, but all of this is happening in a culture where we are building leaders and critical problem-solvers along the way.
> —Gloria Solis, MSN, RN, MBA, NEA-BC, Senior Director of Nursing, The University of Kansas Cancer Center

Kaizen workshops can also include patients as team members to make sure their perspective informs the improvement work in any area. Suppliers and other business partners often participate; their role is the same as everyone else's on the team—to add their expertise to anticipating, identifying, and solving problems.

"When we found that many of our insurance denials were related to eligibility, we invited Experian, our vendor that helps with this digital process, to our Kaizen event," Lasack explained.

Experian sent an expert who participated in the weeklong experience, which included going to the Gemba to help identify where the "pain points" were. Having Experian's perspective on the team generated numerous ideas for improvement.

"Their expert showed us ways to better maximize the use of technology, including adding more payer plans through our query process," Laşack said.

"For the vendor, gaining insight into the complexity of what we're dealing with on the front lines was crucial," added Lasack. "Just bringing the data back to us isn't good enough; it needs to be delivered in a standardized format. If it's understandable and consistent, then we can train to it. Including your business partners in the improvement work can be key to aligning the people, processes, and technology that create better outcomes."

Prove Up

Teams present their work and the outcomes during Friday morning report-out meetings with staff and leaders from across the organization. Page and Peterman are always present. It's an opportunity to make visible what was actually done and the benefit of the work. It also expands organizational learning so others can apply a similar concept or improvement in their area.

Wherever they're in place, Jeff Wright believes the "Lean principles and management system have been transformational."

For the Cancer Center, Kaizen work resulted in 90 percent of "MyChart" patient requests being answered within four hours or less, compared to days or no response at all previously.[12] "In turn, the patients' utilization of this mechanism is going up," Wright confirmed.

MyChart

MyChart	2016*	2017	2018	2019*	Increase/ Improvement
Average Messages/Week	221	295	398	671	204%
Average Patients/Week	127	162	208	327	157%
Median Defect %	14%	11%	13%	9%	35%

*2016 and 2019 are based on partial-year data

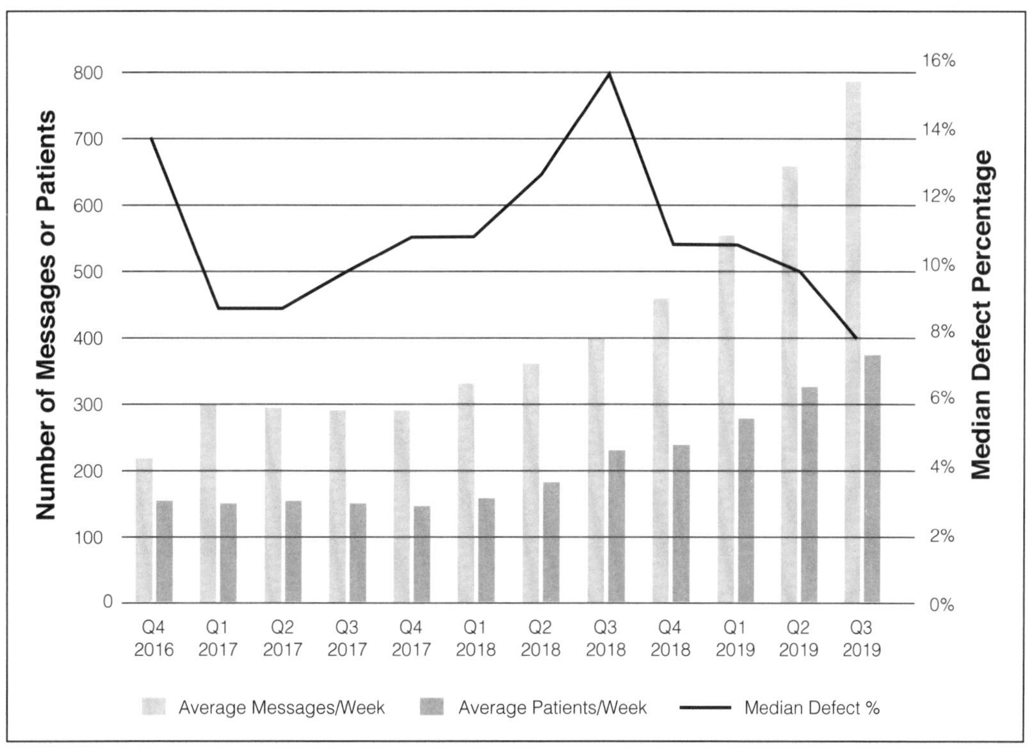

Growing Bigger but Leaner

With over 12,500 employees, the challenge is to make sure that everyone understands Lean and how it applies to every aspect of operations at KU Health System. Doing Lean right is crucial. A census by the Manufacturing Performance Institute indicated that of businesses engaged in Lean initiatives, "74 percent were achieving less than significant results because they weren't implementing it properly."[13] Setting everyone up for success would take training.

That training comes through David Wild's Lean promotion office. There are six defined educational tracks for staff to learn how to support this work in their area.

A series of intense classes, including a written exam, an oral exam, and months of project work, are available "to prove that you are the type of leader who has mastered these concepts and can apply them in your own area," Terry Rusconi explained.

By the end of 2019, over 2,000 members of staff and management had undergone Lean training at KU Health System.

Number of Unique Individuals Involved in Lean Initiatives

Introduction to Lean Tool Workshops:	892
Lean 101 (training):	436
Lean Fundamentals (training):	414
Job Instruction (training):	48
Lean Leadership:	283
Total:	2,073

"With every newly trained employee comes another opportunity to benefit from an empowered staff," Tammy Peterman said.

As efficiencies and innovations are embedded across the organization, achievements are celebrated, and then, from each Kaizen event to the Obeya Room to the units system-wide, the work continues.

For Chris Ruder, RN, COO of the Kansas City Division of KU Health System, the relentless pursuit of improvement isn't about being the best.

"Our most significant competition is not another hospital, health system, industry, or team but what we do not yet internally know," he muses.

CHAPTER SEVEN

Integrate It

[Design] is not just what it looks like and feels like.
Design is how it works.
—Steve Jobs

In 1998, CEOs responding to a survey of 3,700 hospitals across the country reported their second-highest priority was "integrating the delivery system."[1] By 2014, progress on that front was ponderous, with just 31 percent of AMCs nationwide in a process of changing their delivery structure—many were still in discussions about the need to do so.[2] ECG Management Consultants Principal and Head of National Academic Healthcare Christopher Collins, who helped facilitate the integration process at KU Health System, acknowledged that even 31 percent "might have been an overstatement."[3]

For AMCs in particular, the challenge of integrating aspects of health sciences of the university, the faculty practice, and the clinical enterprise is particularly daunting. As The University of Kansas Health System CEO Bob Page put it, "It's hard to get everybody to wear the same jersey."

It's hard to get everybody to wear the same jersey.

At KU Health System, the first conversations about how to affiliate the various players began in 2011. Restructuring the governance and reporting relationships between the university, physicians, and hospital would be no small task operationally or politically. And organizational aspects were only part of the challenge. Each wanted control—especially fiscal control—of its operation. There were complex power issues, consensus-based decisioning struggles, and a lack of accountability between operating units. But the proverbial writing was on the wall: It was critical that the organization find a way to move ahead.

"The success of each AMC component entity is inextricably interdependent," wrote Collins. "The current market can no longer accommodate the disconnect between the hospital, medical school, and faculty practice in areas such as financial and strategic planning."[4]

In a 2014 interview, Dr. Susan Pingleton, former chair of internal medicine at KUMC, described the complicated dynamics, "This is a big family here, but it needs to be happy. We are silos now. We are the university silo, the university physicians silo, the foundation silo, and the hospital silo. To integrate all those silos and have one big silo is what I think of as (clinical) integration."[5]

Those "silos" had been part of a system that had been in place since the 1950s. That system featured 21 separate corporate entities—a state university, the hospital, the physicians' corporation with 18 separate clinical practices—each with its own 501c3 foundation, board, CEO, and checking account. Those foundations had served a purpose.

"They prevented the state from coming in and raiding the accounts of the clinical doctors," explained KU Health System Executive VP of Clinical Affairs and CMO Steve Stites, MD. "So because you're your own company, the state couldn't take your money. All the doctors were employed by those individual companies. I was an employee of the University of Kansas Department of Internal Medicine Foundation. The surgeons were under the General Surgery Foundation. The pathologists were part of the Pathology Foundation, and so on."[6]

As implementation leader for the hospital, I remember the very first meeting we convened; it was not productive. The room was full of multiple representatives from each organization along with their respective lawyers. It may have been one of the most difficult meetings in my career. You could feel the tension; the organizations did not trust each other. But we all seemed to agree on the importance of clinical integration.

We held regular sessions each week—often all-day meetings. About a year into the process, we could feel a trust growing. Negotiations were still difficult, but we had started developing a respect for each other's position.

The mood was professional, but as relationships developed, so did our levity. We were around each other so much, we picked up on one another's mannerisms and habits. At some point, fashion came up, and everyone tried to outdo each other with outlandish socks.

We never lacked for food—I think several of us gained 10 pounds from the cookies and heavy lunches.

Camaraderie developed and kept us diligently moving toward our goal. At some point, we knew we were going to get "there." It took another six months to execute the integration documents (one of the leaders gifted socks to all of us in celebration).

I can honestly say it was the most difficult project of my career, but also the most important and most rewarding.[7]
—William Marting, Former Senior VP and CFO

Beyond Organizational Barriers

For patients, this meant everything from a doctor visit to lab tests to procedures, prescriptions, and billing was subject to varying policies, prices, and processes—even if all services were provided on the same campus. Plus, unique medical records, especially prior to the EMR, were kept for each patient in each department.

"And those were just some of the organizational barriers we had to overcome," said Kirk Benson, MD, VP of clinical integration at KU Health System.

There were a lot of moving parts that needed to work together but "we didn't trust each other," Stites owned. "The hospital was getting all this money while the university and the doctors were taking a hit. There was a lot of bad blood between the hospital, the university, and the physicians' practice."

Indeed, the clinical enterprise at KU Health System was doing remarkably well since its independence from the state system in 1998. With its fiduciary responsibility in mind, restructuring the system both organizationally and functionally was "an immense challenge," according to Benson.

But clinical integration was the culmination of aligning the cost of the clinical enterprise with the mission of the organization; historically, the university was still bearing some of the cost of the clinical enterprise while the hospital really had both the clinical mission and the revenue. Aligning mission and funds flow made sense.

LEADERSHIP LESSON:

Integration is both structural and behavioral.
Both aspects must be addressed.

Page's approach to clinical integration was characteristically deferential: "I'm not the deal guy. I see my role as placing important challenges in front of the organization and letting the right leaders find the best way to make it happen." Leaders stepped forward from all three entities: CFO Bill Marting, SVP Jon Jackson, and general counsel Dan Peters representing the hospital; The University of Kansas Medical Center former Executive Vice Chancellor Doug Girod, MD, and Vice Chancellor of Clinical Affairs Steve Stites, MD, representing the university; and Kirk Benson, MD, president of UKP, and Phil Johnson, MD, chair of radiology, representing the physicians.

"The right people with decision-making authority who could speak truth to one another's power would produce the right outcome," Page said.

Radical Reorganization *without* Crisis

Page and former CEO Irene Thompson had been tasked with generating the necessary tension to compel the changes in 1998 that led to KU Hospital's transformation (see Chapter 1). Indeed, most organizations can't induce substantive change without a crisis forcing their hand, so opting for a radical reorganization in 2012 in the absence of such a crisis was another in a series of unprecedented moves by the health system. It was five years after the hospital had already reached the top 5 percent of AMCs for quality and safety nationwide, a testament to its fully realized transformation. Negative performance wasn't the change agent…a continuous improvement culture was.

"Our path to achieve clinical integration was unique," Benson said. "We proactively chose to undergo the stress of radical organizational changes associated with clinical integration when we were already highly successful."[8]

For KU Health System, the ultimate goal was to provide the highest quality outcomes and best patient experience.

Benson emphasized, "Our leaders had the courage to take us on this path of clinical integration despite our success, knowing it would be disruptive from an individual perspective, and organizationally."

LEADERSHIP LESSON:

Our path to clinical integration was unique because we proactively chose this. We took this on knowing it would be disruptive but necessary to provide an improved, seamless experience for patients.

Differentiating Factors

Proactively initiating clinical integration was in itself a differentiating factor, but KU Health System further antithesized the usual process by completing two major steps at once.

“The biggest headline of the KU Health System story isn’t that the physicians became more aligned with the hospital; it’s that they decided to take two transformational steps simultaneously,” Chris Collins pointed out.[9]

At the outset, Collins had asked them to consider integrating the physicians first, but hands-down, the leadership team said no.

“They insisted that while the sky was not falling, the market would not wait,” Collins recalled. “They wanted to be bold and build a market-leading, highly integrated academic health system in one step.”

To pull that off required synchronizing plans to…

- Wind down 18 individual physician foundations and merge them into a single physician faculty practice plan as a not-for-profit corporation
- Merge the physician group and the teaching hospital/system (TUKHS) and align with KUMC, the university partner

“With regard to the first step, our physician and academic departments each had their own corporate board, and we also had a faculty physician practice plan with a separate board,” Benson explained. “While our academic departments and physicians were successful, our decision-making was slow, and often not aligned. We were wasting limited resources duplicating functions and infrastructure.”

Furthermore, the hospital had its own governing authority board, The University of Kansas Hospital Authority (UKHA), whereas the medical center and university reported to the State Board of Regents. The administrative fragmentation wasn’t doing anything to foster integrated, streamlined decision-making.

LEADERSHIP LESSON:

We were wasting limited resources duplicating functions and infrastructure. We had to move out of the silos and integrate as a system to streamline our operations and stay ahead of the changes in the healthcare industry.

On the university side, they needed cash from the clinical enterprise to keep them afloat, so that was part of the process. The medical school wanted funds from what had become a very successful hospital. This became a driving factor.

I was on some of the committees, and it was a long process. The questions were about who was going to be in charge and how would it work? Compensation plans—how much money would people make; how autonomous were physicians going to be? In orthopedics, we were concerned about the fairness of the non-compete clause.

It wasn't without its bumps, but in the end—with special thanks to Steve Stites and Dan Peters among others—we ended up with a very fair agreement.[10]
—Bruce Toby, MD, Professor and Chair of Orthopedic Surgery

Deliverables

Kirk Benson acknowledged, "It is hard to appreciate the enormity of what our organizations took on to achieve clinical integration."

Benson, Bill Marting, Doug Girod, and Steve Stites led the four-year journey that...

- Phased out 18 distinct clinical corporations that employed the physicians
- Transferred ownership of the legacy physician faculty practice plan (Kansas University Physicians, Inc., i.e., KUPI) to UKHA
- Transferred the 1,000 KUPI clinical and department staff employees to UKHA
- Created a new University of Kansas Physicians (UKP) corporation that would employ the 700+ physician employees transferred from their respective clinical corporations

- Integrated the physician practice plan (UKP) finances into and with TUKHS
- Redesigned the overall governance structure

HOW WE KNOW THAT

Clinical Integration Done Right

Our future depended on our ability to integrate clinical operations. We knew that more functionally integrated AMCs outperformed less integrated health systems, and that would be good for patients. Major changes in the industry—everything from lower reimbursement rates to greater accountability to the Affordable Care Act requirements—basically meant that the demand for more of everything was increasing while the funding to pay for it was decreasing. The opportunity cost of not integrating was having an adverse effect on all three missions that are served by The University of Kansas Health System…and that was a major concern.

When you think about it, an academic health system has three revenue sources. There is the state, and we all know that that's not a very dependable revenue source. Certainly, the academic enterprise gets a lot of money from the state, but that's not something you can rely on forever. Then there are research dollars. Lots of people are chasing that revenue, and I don't think there is going to be a huge abundance of those dollars in the future. So that leaves the clinical dollar.

Ultimately, the clinical/hospital engine drives this campus. That doesn't mean we keep all the clinical dollars in a clinical engine. It means we have to share those dollars with research and education because we are an academic medical center. We're not a community hospital—we have to support all three priorities on this campus.

We approached that goal with physician and hospital leadership oversight just as we'd done with our medical director partnerships. I put a hospital team together that I knew would come back with a proposal for how to do this right.

Trust really had to be in place for this to even begin, so when it got tense or contentious, the commitment and respect between members of that team never wavered.

That was something we had nurtured from the development of medical partnerships and, honestly, looking back, I'd say it just continued to grow.

What I love about this institution is that we did it our way. We didn't follow what they did at XYZ organization; we did what worked in our culture. We knew this had to work, so we took the time to get it right.

With all the contracts in place, we launched on January 1, 2016. The contrast between before and after clinical integration has been like night and day. This has truly been a watershed experience for us.
—Bob Page

LEADERSHIP LESSON:
The clinical engine drives an academic medical center, but that doesn't mean all the clinical dollars remain in the clinical engine. That revenue has to support all three of the missions of an AMC: clinical, research, and education. The most efficient, equitable way to do that is with clinical integration.

Alignment and Cross-Check

Wherever they've been implemented, clinically integrated AMC models are customized to that institution, so there's no one-size-fits-all in the industry. That said, "At KU Health System, we were unique in our approach from the outset," according to Benson. "We developed our model to be fully aligned across our campus, and with our partners. To that end, we have physician and university seats on the governing Health System Board, as well as key System Board Committees."

Those committees, chartered to provide guidance and consultation, touched every aspect of the three missions in which physicians are engaged. They included alignment work across the campus, coordinating the environment for physician practice, and optimizing ambulatory care.

We developed our model to be fully aligned across our campus and with our partners.

These committees focused not just on infrastructural change, but functional changes to ensure doctors would be present and genuinely engaged at the table where decisions got made. A new mission-support model was developed that divvied up revenue based on productivity. The meticulous consideration of each idea took time and extraordinary collaboration.

"They could have said, 'Hey, let's just install a multi-party master agreement as a framework and figure it out over a longer period of time,'" Collins pointed out. "But instead, they leaned into a politically charged environment and crafted a very detailed blueprint with every element predefined before implementation."

They leaned into a politically charged environment and crafted a very detailed blueprint with every element predefined before implementation.

Key Facets of the Integration Model

These key facets are embodied in KU Health System's model:

- Funding: Integrating revenue from physician practices and the clinical enterprise and directing funds to the university in support of the academic agenda. But rather than taking it off the top, as was done in the past, a proportional contribution is tied to the operating margin. In this way, the university's share aligns to the success of the health system. The process is more transparent, accountable, fair, and synergistic.

- Dyad Leadership: Building a dyad management structure of "medical partnership" into strategic ambulatory and hospital-based practices creates direct reporting relationships between the physician practice and the health system executive staff.

"This helps to create and implement standardized clinical and business processes across the enterprise with a focus on optimizing overall performance rather than clinical unit performance," Benson said.

The structure ensures the tripartite mission is considered collaboratively.

"There are times when the focus can be a bit different, but never at the detriment of the other entities," Tammy Peterman said. "We want the leaders of the departments to be autonomous and to be able to make decisions and lead their faculty, but when it comes to the economic and financial expectations, those are shared decisions now as opposed to chairs moving forward with the purchase of something or the hiring of someone. Clinical integration helped us deal with points of contention and work through them. It's created a mechanism for collaboration."

Bruce Toby agreed. "My partner, Charlie Rozanski (vice president, orthopedics and sports medicine), and I have worked well together," he said. "We have a nice relationship and mutual respect."

- Compensation: Paying physicians at market wages was a shared and uncontested priority. This included the hospital absorbing the costs of bringing resident compensation to what the market was paying—also essential in recruiting. Not only did this invigorate competitive hiring, it underscored the clinical commitment to the academic agenda.

  "We are an academic medical center," Bob Page said. "We have researchers on this campus today working on the next breakthrough that will be applied to the patients of tomorrow. So we support each other with that in mind."

In 2016, it was a bold decision to pay physicians at the same rate as their community counterparts rather than at the lower rate traditionally paid by academic medical centers. AMCs don't typically do that. That decision has allowed us to recruit and retain the strongest workforce with outstanding clinical expertise and the best cultural fit.

> We've got the greatest talent from across the country and one of the lowest turnover rates for AMCs. We rarely lose anyone we want to outside organizations. In the end, this has enabled us to achieve exceptional levels of quality, patient satisfaction, and engagement from our medical staff.
> —Steve Stites

- Efficiency: Streamlining processes provides a more seamless experience for the patient. At the beginning of the process, much work was needed.

  "Our clinical departments had developed 23 different practices designed to meet their individual physicians' needs in the complex environment of academic healthcare," explained Keith Sale, MD, associate professor and vice president/chief physician executive, ambulatory services. "Our job was to try and create a unified approach to ambulatory services."[11]

  One of the first initiatives was transitioning electronic scheduling systems to distill over 700 different patient visit types represented in various physician practices into 40 visit types standardized system-wide. Simplifying the incoming patient calls went hand-in-hand with it.

  "We had over 100 different phone numbers that could be called to make an appointment or schedule a procedure," Sale pointed out.

  Establishing one number for each clinical department or division brought this down to fewer than 40.

  Sale added, "Another big win was single-bill. We streamlined so that patients get just one from the health system, not a different kind of bill from the physician, the lab, etc."

Clinical Integration: Before and After Organizational Charts

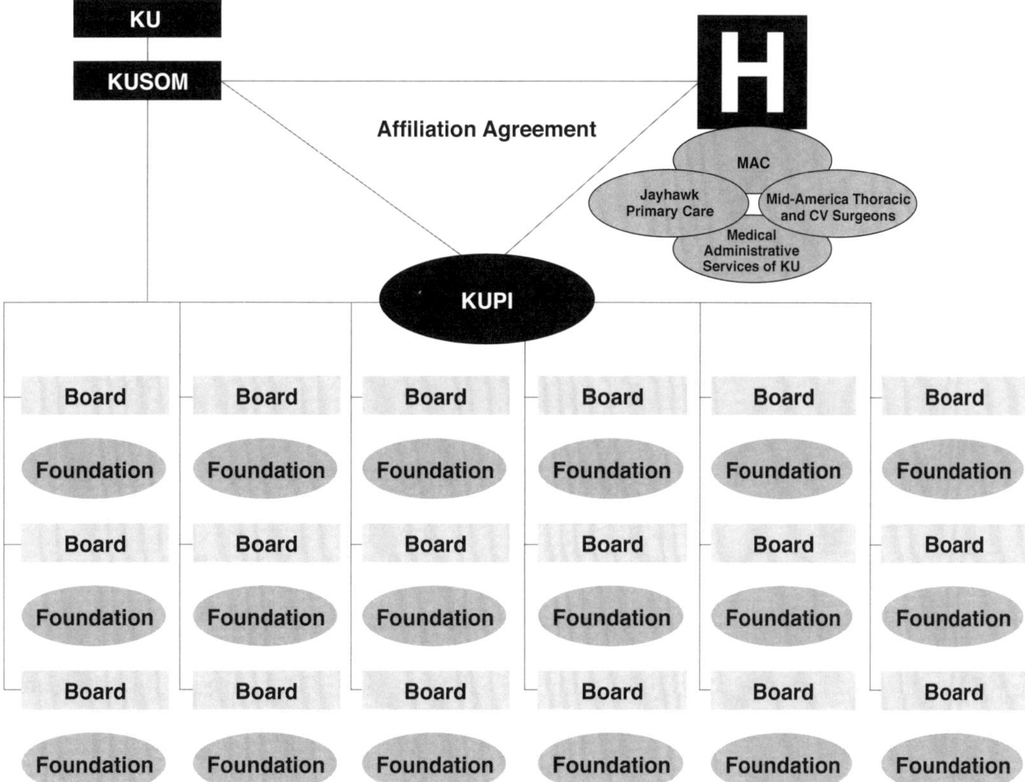

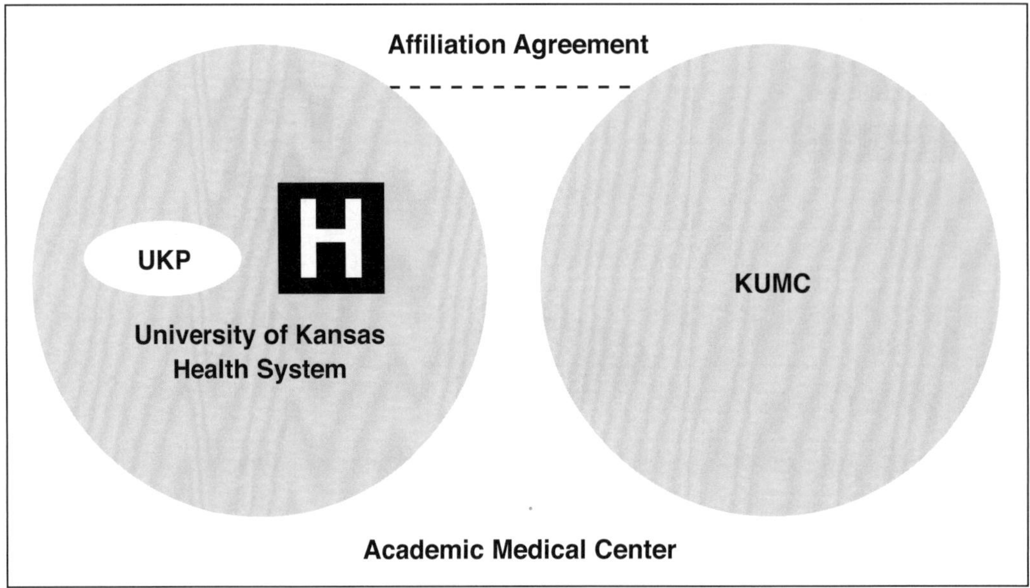

The before and after organizational charts provide a perfect visual for what clinical integration achieved in terms of streamlining and efficiency. It was a colossal, unprecedented effort that set the stage for similar initiatives industry-wide.

"The stuff that has happened here around integration is unlike anything in the country," Steve Stites reflected. "We know that because we keep getting invited to go talk about it."

HOW WE KNOW THAT

Communication, Collaboration, Consistency, and Confidence

We all agreed that a confusing, inconsistent patient experience was a problem we could and must take on. We knew clinical integration could help. And we said if we do this right, it won't matter where you enter the system—every entry point will have streamlined uniformity.

The journey to the legal agreement was an important first step, but the work of creating a truly integrated organization had just begun. The easiest thing to do would have been to continue with the status quo. Yet, for us to achieve everything the system needed from integration, we had to learn how to communicate and collaborate at levels we'd never achieved. And we needed to be consistent in our messages and the way decisions were made, gradually building confidence on the part of everyone involved.

Our most important partners in this work were our clinical service chiefs. They were the leaders of their individual departments and played an essential role in keeping their teams apprised of what was and wasn't happening as a part of clinical integration. We worked tirelessly with them to ensure they were on the front end as topics were being considered and decisions made. They listened and challenged, and we did the same.

We learned it was critical to communicate sooner, not later; to communicate frequently using a wide array of approaches; and to be non-defensive when questions were asked. Years out from clinical integration, we continue to hone these communication channels with our physician partners.

From the outset, we approached clinical integration as a key initiative we were undertaking *along with* our physicians, not something we were *doing to* our physicians. This made collaboration critical to the success of work on which we were embarking.

We created more opportunities for physicians to be involved in board-level work, expanded the medical-director partnerships to engage additional physicians, and fully integrated physicians into the Lean improvement work.

We also began planning strategically and operationally with the department chairs. As essential partners, it was critical we understood their goals and how those could help support the long-term success of the system.

Especially early in the integration journey, consistency was critical—consistency of words to actions, consistency of how each division was engaged in the work being done, and consistency in how decisions were made.

We worked hard with clinical service chiefs and other physician leaders to ensure transparency so they could accurately reflect that consistency to their teams.

This required a great deal of coordinated messaging so everyone had a clear picture of how decisions were made and work was done.
—Tammy Peterman

LEADERSHIP LESSON:
When there's disagreement between parties, it's important to remind yourself (and them) that everyone is on the same team—and then genuinely act accordingly. Be able to articulate the oppositional position and walk a mile in those shoes. Know that the right and sustainable solution is the one that is in everyone's best interests.

Integration with Innovation

In the broadest sense, clinical integration was the penultimate work of partnership. It took the disarray of too many moving parts and made a completely new, highly functional mechanism for serving patients by getting everybody on the same team.

"We're always looking for innovative ways to organize and integrate all of our players more effectively," Bob Page pointed out.

In that same vein, another innovation would engage more players, quite literally, in 2015.

"This organization strives for world-class patient care," explained Shawn Long, VP of corporate and community outreach. "It just follows that we should be the absolute best at everything that's part of this hospital community. When Bob and Tammy brought me on board from the Kansas City Chiefs, they said, 'We have these products and services that businesses need. Let's find ways to partner.'"

At first, Long thought his background in sports sponsorship was a bit of a stretch, but "Bob told me he wanted someone with outside eyes to liaise with corporate partners." Long was given "incredible flexibility to approach this innovatively. It was an idea that's consistent with the culture here—to look at the hospital world a little differently from how the industry usually does."

Hospitals are head down/shoulder into the plow of patient care. To look up and across the horizon for opportunities to serve unmet needs is not how things usually happen in healthcare.

"First, you've got to be looking for those possibilities," Long said. "Second, you've got to have a willingness to explore the entrepreneurial aspects. Bob and Tammy have the right leadership style to authorize that kind of innovation, which takes risk and vision."[12]

Innovating in the Clinical Space

That spirit inspired innovation within the healthcare setting. Through a unique partnership, Kansas City-based Hallmark Cards was able to make its first foray into the hospital gift shop market with a corporate-owned store at TUKHS, a potential new distribution channel for them.

"We've also taken medical experts into the workplace for check-ups or educational workshops for our corporate partners," Long explained. "When we did an on-site skin screening at one location, we identified four of their employees who had something that needed immediate attention. We were able to help them identify that quickly and navigate them through the next steps in their care process."

Many corporate partners have a philanthropic relationship to the hospital, but Long emphasized, "We want to be more than a place to give money. These partnerships help us serve our community in new ways."

It was an idea that's consistent with the culture here—to look at the hospital world a little differently from how the industry usually does.

The corporate partnership innovations have produced:

- The first-ever Hallmark Gold Crown store on-site in a hospital—with community-wide custom-access programs for Hallmark employees.
- A specialized program for executive physicals featuring a personal "navigator" to help executives from companies across the region find what they need from the health system across various campuses and specialties. When a member calls, a navigator provides personal facilitation to the appropriate service or doctor.
- The health system has created a unique sports medicine partnership model with the Kansas City Chiefs, Royals, the T-Mobile (formerly Sprint) Center, and KU Athletics that's focused on ensuring access to cutting-edge care for players, staff, and fans attending events at the various venues. The relationship with KU Athletics, which has been recognized by the NCAA, ensures health system staff oversee all of the trainers, conditioning coaches, and other personnel making decisions about a player's readiness to return to play after an injury.
- As the official healthcare partner of Kansas Speedway, the health system maintains level-one trauma center certification from the American College of Surgeons. This certification meets a requirement established by NASCAR for hosting NASCAR-sponsored races at the speedway. KU Health System also provides all urgent/emergent care for drivers, crew, and fans attending the races.
- KU Health System's focus on sports medicine—including diagnosing and treating concussion—helped inspire the Kansas City Chiefs Fantasy Camp. It was the first of its kind for professional football, providing a once-in-a-lifetime experience for fans. Proceeds help fund the Center for Concussion Management.

LEADERSHIP LESSON:

Corporate partners are more than philanthropic resources; they are a mechanism for healthcare delivery innovation. They help us serve our community in new ways.

Walking into the medical pavilion, the achievement of clinical integration might not be obvious to patients and their families, but another important collaboration is. The aroma of roasted coffee beans draws attention to it in the foyer where The Roasterie Café offers up coffees, pastries, and a model of successfully integrated community partnership at The University of Kansas Health System.

It started humbly back in 1993.

Trying to get his new business off the ground, "I was knocking on doors all day, every day," recalled Danny O'Neill, founder of The Roasterie.[13] The initial purchase of 10 pounds of coffee by KU Hospital launched O'Neill's company, which was just down the road from the health system's main campus. It also fostered the expansion of the hospital's external partnership footprint into community market dynamics in Kansas City.

Today, The Roasterie is a valued vendor for the health system. It donates some of the proceeds from sales of its signature "3901 Blend" (named after what was once the main TUKHS address on Rainbow Boulevard) to the TUKHS-supported employee GED program.

Game On

Partnering with KU Health System has been a boon to the Kansas City Royals, the Chiefs, and The University of Kansas Athletics. In addition to the traditional features of sponsorship, the partnership includes medical care for teams, staff, and fans.

In fact, KU Health System leased about 6,000 square feet that had been unoccupied for years at the Chiefs training complex to provide a clinic complete with X-ray, MRI, and staff, plus additional first aid stations around the stadium.

"Our partnership with TUKHS is based on the trust and understanding of the power created by a mutually beneficial relationship," Kansas City Chiefs President Mark Donovan explained. "In a wide range of areas of our business, the simplest way to say it is they help us win. That's the true impact we all feel."

Kansas City Royals GM Dayton Moore concurred.

"Our entire organization—players, staff, and even families—have benefited greatly from our relationship with The University of Kansas Health System," said Moore. "Our ability to utilize the expertise of their incredible doctors and staff has, without a doubt, given us a competitive advantage within Major League Baseball."

LEADERSHIP LESSON:

It takes an entrepreneurial outlook to find new ways to fill unmet healthcare needs. Innovation in the clinical space and patient services delivered off-site become creative ways to fully engage in your organizational mission.

Teaming with the big leagues has had ancillary benefits.

"Across the Midwest, this health system is well known, but people in San Diego or New York are often unaware of our outcomes, our NCI-designation, or our national ranking," Long explained. "Our external partnerships with sports teams show a level of trust and credibility that's getting national attention."

It's not just about the face of healthcare today—it's about its legs. We're finding ways to bring our services to the places where people work and live in our community.

While national attention isn't the goal, it is a by-product of external partnership. And external partnerships also help deliver the mission of KU Health System "as an academic health system serving the people of Kansas, the region, and the nation," said Bob Page.

"It's not just about the face of healthcare today—it's about its legs," Page continued. "Being willing and able to innovate with our community partners means we're finding ways to bring our services to them. This promotes healthier workplaces and more convenient access to healthcare for employees."

At The University of Kansas Health System, innovation and integration work in tandem—one without the other doesn't reach the goal. Together, they coalesce in a culture of excellence and continuous improvement. "It's all about applying the best of what we know so we can advance this health system to higher levels," Bob Page says.

CHAPTER EIGHT

Advance It

Progress lies not in enhancing what is, but in advancing toward what will be.
—Khalil Gibran

Three hours earlier, the patient had been talking and joking with staff in his hospital room, but now he was in critical condition on a ventilator in the ICU. Especially during the early months of the pandemic, the "battle routine"—as KU Health System caregivers would come to call the rigid protective procedures and rapid diligence with COVID-19 patients—wasn't even routine yet. But the pandemic was surging, and it was a battle—one patient at a time.

Since family members couldn't be present in the room during the lockdown stage, doctors and nurses were often the only people there to hold up an iPad or notebook so patients could communicate with family at home and provide updates.

"We had to spend a lot of time physically in the room via Skype or Zoom getting families the information they needed," said Chris Brown, MD, an internal medicine physician at The University of Kansas Health System.

Brown reflected on what it was like to be on the front lines in a personal video diary.

"The true impact on the nursing staff, medical students, respiratory therapists, and other direct care workers—environmental services, food services, everybody—I did not know the toll this would take on this healthcare system," Brown admitted. "*Thank you* just isn't enough."[1]

His video joined many others that were uploaded to the health system's intranet so staff could share their experiences to stay grounded and gain emotional support.

Whether it's an innovation on a personal level supporting weary patients, physicians, and staff; or providing cutting-edge medicine and healthcare delivery; or stepping up with leadership to the community and beyond, advancing the cause of this health system takes many forms.

One of those forms prompted a small-town reporter with the *Wichita Eagle* to contact KU Health System for the same reason a CNN producer did. Both wanted access to the Medical News Network and broadcast studio *STAT* for an interview with an expert on COVID-19.

Both came to the same right place.

LEADERSHIP LESSON:

In the age of the pandemic, a world-class healthcare organization has a role and a responsibility to the global community.

Leadership Lessons from the Pandemic

In response to a global pandemic, I am proudest of our ability to rapidly evolve and adapt from a system level down to the individual patient level. We shifted protocols and processes of internal functioning to optimally address the needs of our caregivers and patients—almost on a dime.

Locally, we led the way in diagnostics, therapeutics, and infection prevention and control of COVID-19. Although we've had systems in place for new and emerging infections and pathogens, we were able to quickly obtain in-house testing and develop further protocols and systems specifically related to this virus to keep our patients and healthcare workers safe during evaluation and treatment.

KU Health System also led the collaboration with other area hospitals to learn what was going on in our region, and coordinate our efforts and messages to the public about the current state of the disease in this community.

In my opinion, we've done a major service in educating the public regionally and even nationally with our live newscast of daily media briefings on the current state of crisis and its impact. We focused on the best way for people to protect themselves and their loved ones while also providing accurate, up-to-date information about the disease process and therapeutics. Patients who had recovered, nurses and physicians on the front lines, political leaders, and specialists brought many perspectives to the dialogue. And we stressed the importance of not neglecting chronic diseases. People needed reassurance about seeing their healthcare providers and how to re-enter society safely.

The takeaways for the industry at large include the utmost importance of training of personnel. Training must be available and reinforced for our caregivers so they perform optimally and remain healthy in order to care for our patients. Additionally, having adequate stores of materials and critical drugs for patient care is crucial. Maintaining that supply chain is vitally important to any operation.

On that note, here's my last lesson: People want to help…let them. We were contacted by so many individuals offering goods and services, such as making masks for our employees on their sewing machines and businesses with digital printing services making face shields. Large companies donated time and services, including alcohol sanitizer and meals for our people working on the front lines every day.

We live in an amazing place, and it was so inspiring to see everyone—inside this health system and outside in our community—rise to meet this challenge.
—Dana "Hawkeye" Hawkinson, MD, Infectious Diseases/Medical Director of Infection Prevention and Control, MNN Morning Media Update Co-Host

In an era of pandemic health threats, "A world-class healthcare organization has a role and a responsibility to the global community," says Bob Page. "Everything we've learned about patient-centered care provides an opportunity to advance the cause we serve."

The News Everyone Needs

When The University of Kansas Health System launched the "Medical News Network" (MNN) in 2014 out of its sleek, new, state-of-the-art Dolph C. Simons, Jr., Family Broadcast Studio, it had two goals:

- To provide an exclusive newsfeed to journalists of the most current healthcare and medical information
- To be the first-of-its-kind hospital-based studio to use LTN cloud-based fiber optics—the same system CNN was adopting—to link directly to cable and television networks anywhere in the world

> We've regarded The University of Kansas Hospital as a shining example of forward-thinking and commitment to excellence. As a newspaper family, we recognize how important it is to make information available to the public and to provide expertise to put new developments in perspective...this studio can do something to help KU Hospital continue to be a more recognized leader.
> —Dolph C. Simons, Jr.

The MNN approach was so novel that it would eventually be trademarked for "First Use to The University of Kansas Hospital Authority."[2] Whereas other in-house studios at the Mayo Clinic or Baylor were focused on patient education and internal communications, MNN was broadcasting to the world.

"Advancing healthcare means sharing what we've learned as widely as possible—our Medical News Network is an important vehicle for that," Tammy Peterman affirmed.

From medical breakthroughs to topical health and wellness information, cutting-edge research, interviews with physicians and subject experts, and compelling patient profiles, the content volume is matched only by the accessibility of MNN. And the MNN studio also has LIVE capabilities for breaking news and a host of other interactive applications.

"We don't write their stories for them, but we do provide 'raw' HD 1080i video and MP3 files that reporters can use to create their own news stories," explained Jill Chadwick, TUKHS media relations and news director. This unprecedented resource is tapped 24/7 by journalists locally and internationally.

Take-10

At the onset of COVID-19, we agreed to "live by" several communication principles:

- We need to connect with one another.
- In times of uncertainty, we will help staff/patients gain some control by giving them knowledge.
- Employees must feel safe; employees who feel safe will help patients feel safe.
- We will be transparent/create trust.
- What we say inside the organization will be communicated outside whether we like it or not, so let's use this fact to our advantage.
- We will be leaders.

Created at the beginning of the pandemic, "Take-10" became an integral tool in our communication process. It's a ten-minute intranet broadcast we produce from our in-house studios. It features Bob Page and Tammy Peterman speaking directly to staff about what's happening—everything from safety and PPE information to changes in the supply chain to how our physical environment is being altered to meet patient needs. Employees can start the day with these 6:30 a.m. updates from our executive leadership every Monday through Friday.

From its beginnings, the Take-10 video format allowed Bob and Tammy to speak directly to employees across our facilities in a way that previously hadn't been possible because of our size and the limitations imposed by the pandemic. The quick in-and-out format was convenient for sharing and receiving information, and for building confidence that executive leadership was aware of what staff at the bedside and working from home were facing.

> Because Take-10 has been an effective way to reach employees across our system, we've continued it daily, and have rotated in additional executive leaders several times each week.
> —Gayle Sweitzer, VP of Marketing and Corporate Communications

In the early days of the COVID-19 pandemic, MNN began broadcasting the "Morning Media Update," a live, interactive newscast every Monday through Friday co-hosted by Chief Medical Officer and Executive Vice President of Clinical Affairs Steve Stites, MD, and Dr. Dana Hawkinson, medical director of infection prevention and control. It was picked up by CNN and livestreamed by other news agencies nationwide, achieving 10,998,075 total impressions—national and international. The broadcast and digital news reach grew to 2.45 billion in just the first six weeks of its broadcast.[3]

Viewers could pose their questions on the topic for live, interactive response from the featured physicians, frontline caregivers, recovered patients, hospital leadership, and elected officials.

The second time U.S. Senator for Kansas Jerry Moran participated, he joined remotely via satellite link from studios in the U.S. Capitol Building in Washington DC. Moran quickly became a regular Friday morning guest to provide federal insight on available aid programs, PPE supplies, and a national perspective. The MNN broadcast studio technology worked seamlessly with its DC counterpart, proving itself an effective, timely mechanism for communication between Senator Moran and folks back home.

Not only is this a valuable thing for Kansas City, but it's being seen nationwide as the standard for how to communicate and share information. Love leading from the heartland!

The viability of this live, interactive exchange wasn't lost on legislators from other states.

"I've had multiple Senate offices reaching out and asking me how we are coordinating this, because they're trying to replicate it in their states," said Tom Brandt, communications director for Senator Jerry Moran. "Not only is this a valuable thing for Kansas City, but it's being seen nationwide as the standard for how to communicate and share information. Love leading from the heartland!"[4]

"We view it this way," Page explained. "*To lead the nation in caring, healing, teaching, and discovering* is not just our mission statement; it's our marching orders."

LEADERSHIP LESSON:
To lead the nation in caring, healing, teaching, and discovering is not just our mission statement; it's our marching orders.

Marching Side by Side: Academics and Clinical Care

The Medical News Network serves as a beacon for the groundbreaking work being done at TUKHS. There is arguably no better place to advance the best practice of healthcare than an academic medical center that joins research to clinical practice. There's a long history of pioneering collaboration at KU Health System including what may have been the very first "medical director partnerships" in the nation.[5]

Today, formalized, strategically linked, and goal-driven medical partnerships are in place across the country, but they may have actually had their genesis at The University of Kansas Hospital in the '90s. At that time, the chairs' structure was academically focused and didn't play an active role in the clinical agenda. Former CEO Irene Thompson had been looking for ways to break through that structural barrier and engage doctors from the medical school with the emerging clinical agenda of KU Hospital. As she recalled, "It was nearly impossible to get physicians to attend meetings called by the hospital."

The idea of establishing financially supported partnerships between medical and clinical directors—who could be department heads, nurse managers, or other leaders across the clinical enterprise—created a necessary mechanism for collaboration and innovation at a time when the clinical chairs were not fully engaged in this work. Thompson acknowledged, "I don't know that we were recognized for it. We presented it at the University

HealthSystem Consortium and IHI's Quality Management Network, and many there adopted it."[6]

LEADERSHIP LESSON:

Create mechanisms for collaboration—starting with physicians and administrators and continuing until everyone identifies as a member of a team.

After full implementation, Thompson was relieved to find "the attitude changed. There was standing room only at the routine luncheon meeting of these partnerships to discuss improvements that were being made."

Formalizing partnerships had created a mechanism for collaboration—starting with physicians and administrators.

Thompson acknowledged, "It was a notable innovation."

And that innovation would have far-reaching effects.

Disrupting the SOP

An additional benefit of the novel medical/clinical director partnerships was the disruption of the historically precedented "doctor said/nurse did" standard operating procedure. Since medical director partnerships were non-hierarchal by design, "These partnerships engaged physicians and nurse managers as true collaborators," Tammy Peterman explained.

As a standard operating procedure, "Determining a patient's plan of care had always been the physician's turf, but with the medical director partnerships, nursing input was elevated," she added. "Nurses were right there seeing what worked best for the patient. Their insights were incorporated in ways that improved the patient's clinical progress and care experience. That couldn't be discounted."

Teaming doctors and nurses on an equal level "incubated relationships, developed skillsets, and advanced our organizational strength," Terry Rusconi confirmed. "What we nurtured 20 years ago was a foundation that's still supporting the collaborative way medicine is practiced here."

LEADERSHIP LESSON:

Teaming doctors and nurses on an equal level incubates relationships, develops skillsets, and advances organizational strength.

Medical director partnerships evolved with outcomes in mind.

"Instead of medical directors getting paid ipso facto just for showing up with their title, we said, 'Show us the project you're working on with your clinical partner,'" explained Steve Stites, MD, executive VP of clinical affairs and chief medical officer. "'Write it up and complete it. When you're done, we're going to help you publish so you can disseminate what's been learned.'

"That's how the medical partnership model works now," he added. "A team can submit a proposal around quality or financial improvement, and if it's approved, the health system partner and a physician are bringing their expertise together toward a common goal."

All medical director partnerships must:

- Engage physicians in the development of and improvement to patient care practices.
- Encourage innovation and teamwork to solve problems effectively from both physician and administrative perspectives.
- Provide an opportunity for both physician and clinical director to learn operational and leadership skills to support them in their career growth.

Theory to Practice

Medical partnerships proved their mettle early on with the development of a ventilator-weaning protocol in 1999. A group of partnerships, including medical directors of surgery, medicine ICU, respiratory therapy, and ICU nurse managers, collaborated on strategies to help respiratory therapists get patients off breathing support as quickly as possible. They developed, got approved, and implemented a protocol that required a team approach to weaning the patient off the ventilator without the need for an additional physician order.

This reduced the risk of the patient's developing ventilator-associated pneumonia, a significant side effect of prolonged intubation, while decreasing length of ICU stay, reducing reintubation, and lowering costs. The protocol has been standard operating procedure at KU Health System ever since.

The protocol has been standard operating procedure at KU Health System ever since.

In 2014, another medical partnership group, including the medical directors, hospital directors, and other staff from Trauma/Critical Care and the Surgical Intensive Care Unit, engaged in a project that produced even more profound results. The partnership implemented a spontaneous awakening trial (SAT) with mechanically ventilated, sedated ICU patients. The goals included reducing sedation usage and days, ICU days, ventilator utilization, and mortality.

The results were both dramatic and surprising. Five units experienced a decrease in sedation usage, and all seven units experienced an improvement in mortality index from baseline. The risk-adjusted mortality index went from underperforming the UHC top performer benchmark by 0.15 in the first year of the study to outperforming that same benchmark by 0.15 at the end of the third year.[7]

Cost Savings from SAT[8]

Reduced Sedation Usage	$ 93,600
Reduced Length of Stay	$ 817,412
Reduced Ventilator Days	+ $ 758,928
Total Impact	$ 1,669,940

"Reduced sedation days translate to more days the patients are awake and participating in their care," Lynelle Pierce, RN, MS, CCRN, CCNS, FAAN, said. "The hallmarks of medical partnerships in our collaborative culture—data-driven analysis, application of best-known practices, and development of new best practices—are what enable initiatives like this to happen."

All seven units experienced an improvement in mortality index from baseline.

Such collaboration is still very much in the works today. Structure for the partnership is built into the process. Medical and hospital director partners meet regularly to discuss ongoing work and status of projects. Updates are shared at partnership group meetings, monthly luncheons, clinical chair and medical staff meetings, and with executive leadership.

Physician VP for Perioperative and Procedural Services Sean Kumer, MD, and Lila Martin, VP of Perioperative Services (at the time), were medical partners between 2017 and 2018. "Our new 'North Stars' are not only to improve the efficiency of the OR and enhance the patient experience, but we hope to improve our employee satisfaction in a cost-conscious and effective manner," Kumer explained. "We always place the patient front and center, which is paramount. To paraphrase a Richard Branson quote, *If you ensure that your employees are happy, then they will always ensure that your patients are happier.* We want the best outcome for our patients always, so why shouldn't we also strive for the same expectations for our employees?"

Perioperative & Procedural Services: Medical Partnership Wins[9]

- Increased the number of cases performed in same duration of time despite no increases in OR space/rooms
- Decreased the total amount of time between patient arrival and case completion by eliminating waits and ensuring the efficiency of systems and processes to safely prepare the patient for surgery
- Increased the number of first case on-time starts (FCOTS)

- Decreased the time necessary to prep the patient prior to going to surgery by streamlining the handoffs between various clinicians involved in the process
- Decreased turnover time between cases
- Increased the safety of the patients' experiences with improved timeouts and involvement of the entire surgical team in safety and equipment discussions
- Eliminated the risk of lost or misplaced OR specimens by standardizing processes and ensuring effective documentation of handoffs
- Decreased cancellation rates by enhancing/standardizing the pre-op evaluations

LEADERSHIP LESSON:

We've learned that collaboration and innovation can and should be structured and supported—not simply encouraged. Our medical director partnerships have produced many of our most successful initiatives.

Medical partnerships became an important strategy to promote a mutually invested process.

"We started with about 10 partnerships that blossomed into somewhere between 80 and 100. So many successful initiatives on this campus are the outcome of a medical director partnership," Tammy Peterman pointed out. "And the partnerships are producing outcomes that influence operations throughout our entire health system. Unit 62 is the 'model cell' for inpatient care. Their medical director partnership has produced incredible outcomes that we're replicating system-wide."[10]

A Model Medical Partnership

When Dr. Matt Jones walks into KU Hospital's Medicine/Telemetry Unit, a.k.a., Unit 62, he leaves his title at the door.

"From the 'hello' from the unit nurse at the welcome desk to the high-five on the floor, you're noticed, you're greeted, it feels like home," says Jones, DO, internist and assistant professor at KUMC. "It's a great feeling to be rounding up here. They're all so good at what they do, you know your patients are going to be taken care of; you have trust."

When her medical director partnership began with Jones in 2016, Tori Butler, RN, was nurse manager of Unit 62, the bellwether of acute-care best practice at KU Health System.

"This unit is considered a model cell, because every new idea tested here will be implemented system-wide if we demonstrate success and sustainability," Butler explained. "But what we've found with system-wide spread is it works only if you have the right culture and daily management system to go with it."

LEADERSHIP LESSON:

What we've discovered about implementing a great idea system-wide is that it works only if you have the right leadership and culture to support and sustain it.

One of the first projects they collaborated on involved best practice rounding with a workshop called "Physician Day of Care."

"Initially, this was very unit-driven," Butler said. "The nursing team and I would focus on specific things with each physician who rotated on this unit. We provided background information on the specific metrics and goals of daily rounds, discussed questions, did reminders during huddles, and then followed-up with outcomes to each doctor at the end of that week. I would trend the progress and outcomes and send to each provider weekly along with various leadership and interdisciplinary team members.

"Over time, the data showed statistically significant impact when this practice was consistently followed," she explained.[11] "We really worked hard to remove the pebbles from the physicians' shoes to get buy-in and make this successful."

Physicians want to do the right thing, but are sometimes unaware of changes that become necessary between their rounds. Nurses help by providing information and insight.

"Nurses are the 'why' behind my 'ask,'" Dr. Matt Jones said. "Nurses are going to come talk to you if there's an issue—they'll bring it up directly."

Tori Butler, RN, observes this daily with her staff.

"Our nurses will examine a process or scenario with a doc and play catch-ball with ideas to see if there's a better way," she said. "We've seen firsthand how this leads to better outcomes."

Keeping It Real

For Jones and Butler, the definition of medical partnership is about having mutual goals, focus, and respect.

"I don't feel as though I have to agree with Matt because he's a physician," Butler said. "My input and position on things are equal to his, even though he's a physician. This is rare, but it's necessary—we can disagree and have a conversation about why."

LEADERSHIP LESSON:

The best dynamic between doctors and nurses is one where each respects the other's role and expertise. Our nurses will examine a process or scenario with a doc and play catch-ball with ideas to see if there's a better way.

Jones agrees.

"We can be real; we don't beat around the bush," he says. "I'll push back on her; she will on me. We get better at managing conflict and working in partnership. Knowing that we have the same goal in mind, and respect for each other and the whole team, I don't have to worry about how Tori is representing us in the various places she reports out—it's exactly how I'd be thinking. Or if it isn't, I trust that I'll understand her perspective when we process the idea later. We both grow from that in our expertise and as a team."[12]

My input and position on things are equal to his, even though I'm a nurse. This is rare, but it's necessary—we can disagree and have a conversation about why.

Their medical partnership benefits from their collegiality, but also because the KU Health System culture encourages this model.

"It's not about me as nurse manager, but about collaboration and leadership," Butler said, with Dr. Jones adding, "Servant leadership."

It Takes Two: The Dyad Model

Recognizing the value of partnerships, collaboration and leadership were reflected in a new, expanded leadership structure that strengthened physician roles on the executive team in 2018. Executive leadership dyads were created by formally partnering a physician leader with an administrative leader to manage selected aspects of business.

The dyad approach expanded to include triad leadership as well. For example, day-to-day management of the health system's ambulatory services practice is overseen by a triad consisting of a physician executive, a nurse executive, and an administrative executive. Additional dyads comprised of senior administrators and department chairs focus on the administrative and clinical operation of that particular department/division.

LEADERSHIP LESSON:

To do this right, we have to think about systems and physician practice simultaneously.

A unique role for physicians grew out of this model.

"People who are in the business of medicine do not always speak the same language as those people who practice the art of medicine," said Keith Sale, MD, associate professor at KUMC and vice president and chief physician executive of ambulatory services. "As physician leaders in the dyad leadership model, we are the translators filling in the gaps and connecting the dots. That's our role. We try really hard to be advocates for our peers and partners. We have to think about systems and physician-practice simultaneously."

In 2019, KU Health System's collaboration model subsumed all non-executive physician partnership programs into what would be called the "Care Connections Partnership Program."

Great Moments in Medical Partnership

Director of Rehabilitation Services Julie Ginter and Sarah Eickmeyer, MD, Acute Inpatient Rehabilitation Unit medical director, teamed up on numerous projects, including a successful initiative to reduce hospital readmissions to their department that brought that figure down from 14.8 percent to 8.7 percent.[13]

"Julie and Sarah exemplify what we're trying to do with this program," says Dorothy McGhee, director of special projects at The University of Kansas Health System. "They have good communication. They set goals, collaborate, and achieve outcomes that reflect well on their objectives."

Focusing on patients who become ill during acute inpatient rehab and have to be readmitted, Ginter and Eickmeyer established a performance improvement project goal to decrease the acute-care readmission rate to less than 10 percent within a six-month period. Data review from August 2014 to January 2015 identified a readmission rate of 14.8 percent and sepsis as the most common cause. In collaboration with unit nursing leadership, they developed training to improve patient monitoring and communication, modified the admissions process, increased unit resources, and facilitated changes to the electronic medical record (EMR).

After implementation, the overall readmission rate from the rehab unit back to acute care decreased from 14.8 percent to 8.7 percent.

"We were pleased. The results indicated that appropriate interventions can reduce readmission rates," Eickmeyer said.

Reducing Acute-Care Readmissions: The Components of an Intervention Strategy

Education/Communication

- Half-day seminar for healthcare provider education
- Information session for onboarding residents
- Adoption of "ISBARR" RN-MD communication tool
- "Badge Buddy" (concise patient management instructions) provided to RN

Admission/Process Modifications

- Checklist to review stability of patients prior to admission
- Implementation of formal handoff between discharging acute hospital physician and admitting rehabilitation resident physician
- Continued IV/central line access at time of admission

Unit Resources

- Increased availability of commonly administered IV antibiotics
- RN training to use ultrasound for IV catheter insertion
- Creation of overnight nurse unit coordinator position

Electronic Medical Record (EMR) Modifications

- Revision of order set to include pertinent orders for declining patients
- Improved functionality with assistance of IT (e.g., improved presentation of data in flowsheets)

This multi-factored intervention exemplifies the best of collaboration via the medical director partnership.

"Part of what makes this successful is that Sarah is an exceptional physician when it comes to open communication," said Ginter. "She's patient-focused, programmatic, and staff-centered—all qualities that help us be successful. The relationship is trusting and responsive."

"It's easy to have a good relationship because our goals are aligned," Eickmeyer adds. "We have an easy partnership because we both want the same thing for our program and our patients."

Advancing the Care Connection

The Care Connection categorized the health system's collaborative projects by type:

- **Regulatory Partnerships** as required by accrediting, regulatory, or governing bodies. Following the traditional model, these directors were identified through a collaborative process between the hospital and the clinical chairs and compensated based on a fixed number of hours per month.
- **Administrative Partnerships** as required by the health system to provide a necessary administrative function. These directors were also identified through a collaborative process between the hospital and the clinical chairs with compensation based on a fixed number of hours per month.
- **Care Advancement Partnerships** opened up an application process for teams to focus on clinical or outcomes improvement as directed by the health system's strategic initiatives. The partners could submit a proposal detailing the idea, projecting the amount of time needed, and providing the names of the physician and health system partner for consideration by an executive steering committee. As many projects as can be funded are chosen for the care advancement partnerships. Compensation for these partnerships is based on the completion of the project.

It also modified the compensation model. Compensation for the dyad partners was based on completing a project, not logging time. From a continuous improvement perspective, this approach emphasized outcomes. "All work is incentivized and compensated in alignment now, and focused on completion," David Wild, MD, vice president of performance improvement, pointed out. "We built a lot of process into that to help teams build realistic, achievable goals."[14]

"We heard from our early- to mid-career physicians that they wanted more opportunities to develop leadership skills and impact organizational performance," Terry Rusconi said.

The care advancement partnerships leveraged into career advancement nicely.

The Care Collaborative

One of the most important tools for advancing healthcare at KU Health System wasn't a medical breakthrough but, quite literally, a car. Specifically, the "CareCar." This mobile clinic emerged from an effort to reach patients in some of the remotest regions of the state out of KU Health System's "Care Collaborative."

"We applied for and received a $12.5 million challenge grant from the Centers for Medicare & Medicaid Services in 2014," Tammy Peterman said. "I think it was the eighth largest grant CMS awarded in that round. The goal was to improve the health of heart attack and stroke victims, and explore cost-efficient solutions for healthcare in rural areas."

KU Health System teamed Bob Moser and Jodi Schmidt, a physician and an administrator respectively, to lead the effort into central and western Kansas.

Our focus on rural acute care was to get everyone in agreement on evidence-based guidelines, and then to adopt them.

The CareCar

With all the digitalization of medical equipment, Greg Thomas, a professor at the KU School of Architecture and Design, was interested in how this technology could be put to use in a mobile clinic. He envisioned a miniature van with modular equipment—anything from a clinic that could be loaded into a specially designed suitcase and brought to a remote site. He had been looking for some organization to put this theory into practice, so when we heard about Greg's idea at The University of Kansas Health System, we said, *Hey, we can do this tomorrow!*

We went straight to work. Our plan called for deploying the mobile clinic or "CareCar" cross-country doing "house calls" on patients shortly after they had been discharged home following a heart attack or stroke. Those patients were either served on-site, referred on to an appropriate specialist, or discharged as necessary. The CareCar visited patients in all kinds of settings, even rural senior housing environments to reach patients who'd been going without care or meds.

Everywhere we've been created a great opportunity to find out what works or what doesn't. And what we've learned from rural areas, we've subsequently moved into the Kansas City metro area, and now we're trying those ideas in an urban setting.[15]
—Bob Moser, Physician Executive Advisor, Care Collaborative
—Jodi Schmidt, Executive Director, Care Collaborative

Initially known as the "Kansas Heart and Stroke Collaborative," the Care Collaborative project included KU Health System, the HaysMed campus, and 11 critical access hospitals across 13 counties in northwest Kansas. Moser and Schmidt implemented the acute-care arm of the project and two ambulatory arms.

"Our focus on acute care was to get everyone in agreement on evidence-based guidelines for heart care/stroke and adopting practices for rural communities," Schmidt explained. At 13 hospitals in the region, "Everyone signed on and developed protocols for managing heart attack and stroke. Then our staff went out to establish baseline measures."

Baseline indicators showed the percentage of patients receiving the necessary drugs to treat their acute condition was well below national average. As a result, the hospitals were never able to do even the first steps in the evidence-based care bundle. Given that national research studies showed it can take a decade for research to become practice, the Kansas Heart and Stroke Collaborative bucked the trend entirely.

"We were able to help them do this in months instead of years," Schmidt affirmed. "We measured change from before to after training, and we showed that we were able to move the needle that quickly. Dr. Moser is too modest to point this out, but it's true."

Care Collaborative Quality Performance Measures[16]

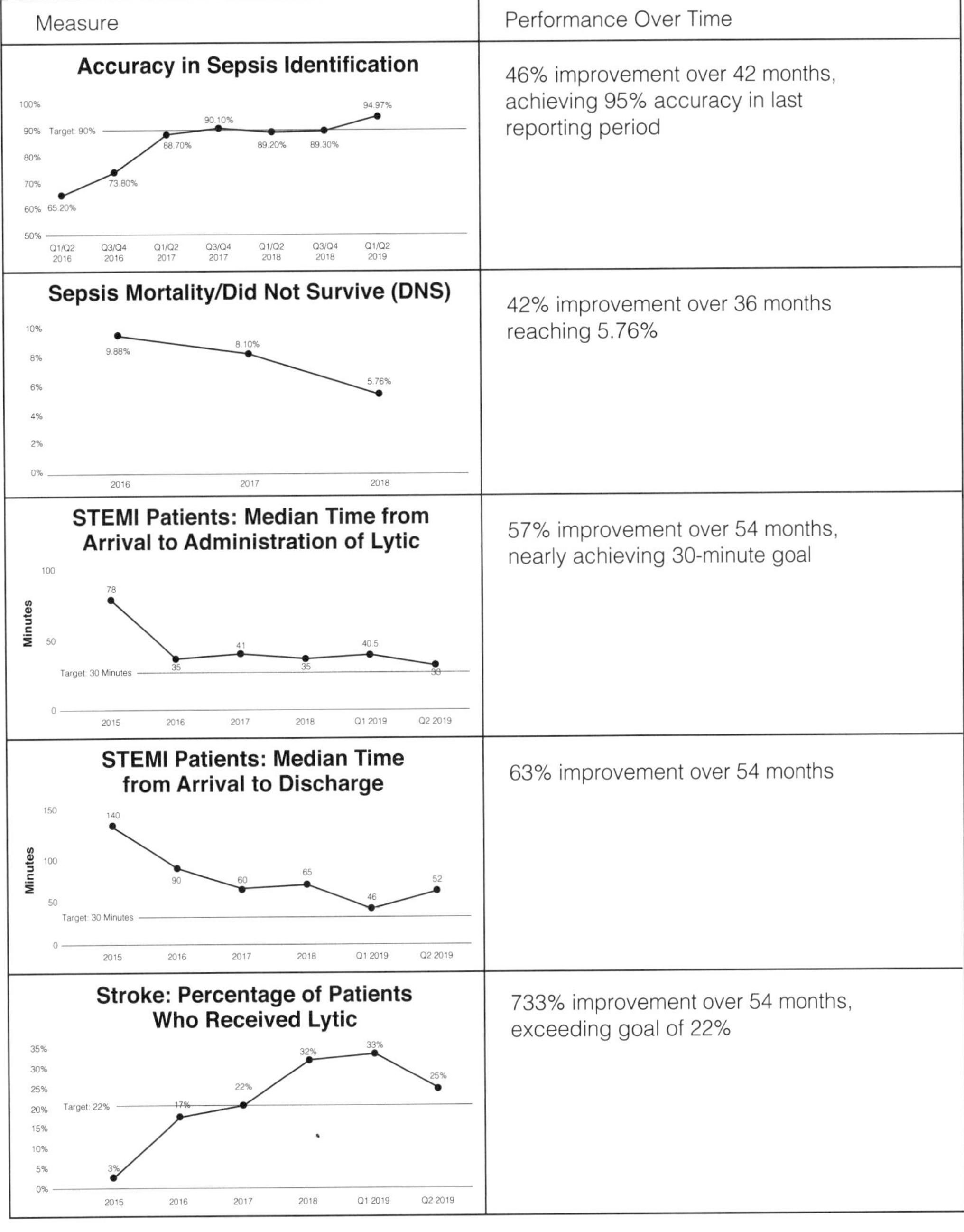

Measure	Performance Over Time
Accuracy in Sepsis Identification	46% improvement over 42 months, achieving 95% accuracy in last reporting period
Sepsis Mortality/Did Not Survive (DNS)	42% improvement over 36 months reaching 5.76%
STEMI Patients: Median Time from Arrival to Administration of Lytic	57% improvement over 54 months, nearly achieving 30-minute goal
STEMI Patients: Median Time from Arrival to Discharge	63% improvement over 54 months
Stroke: Percentage of Patients Who Received Lytic	733% improvement over 54 months, exceeding goal of 22%

What Moser will say is, "We had a great team, and we had excited and willing rural providers. Both Jodi and I have a history in rural healthcare, and we understood the challenges they were facing. They don't always have the time even if they do have the desire. There's such a broad scope of their practice. It falls to them to try to do everything. They greatly appreciated this connection back to the AMC so they could use best practices."

LEADERSHIP LESSON:

Rural healthcare providers have a broad scope of practice, but instead of feeling overwhelmed by "one more thing to do," they welcomed the training that enabled them to stay abreast of best practices. Improving the quality of care is possible anywhere providers are supported with the knowledge and tools—especially in rural communities.

Both Moser and Schmidt credit the project's success to the local providers who were highly invested in it. One CNO told Schmidt she wanted to know all she could about best practices, but staying abreast of evidence-based medicine is challenging in a rural setting. For her, the collaborative support "made it easy."

The Care Collaborative went on to cover not only heart attack and stroke, but sepsis, heart failure, and palliative/end-of-life care across 66 counties. Training on evidence-based protocols and best practices is provided in each community, but Moser acknowledged, "We merely assist them in adapting the protocols and implementing best practices for their local realities based on the resources or circumstances they face. We focus on what we can help them accomplish through data-driven performance improvement."

Providers, nursing, lab, and other staff as well as local long-term care folks can participate in one of two training sessions offered on one day to cover all shifts of the hospital.

Moser said, "Doing this ensures everyone in the local health system is trained on their organization's adopted protocols at the same time."[17]

For Moser, the work is incredibly satisfying.

"I trained here and practiced on the Kansas/Colorado border for 25 years," he said. "I didn't think KU Health System knew I existed out here, so I really appreciate what I'm doing now. It's a win/win."

Schmidt concurred.

"CEOs would say to me, 'I can't ask my people to do one more thing now, Jodi,' but their team would tell them, 'No, no! We want this! We need this!!'" he said. "It's been so gratifying—working with people who want what you're providing."

I trained here and practiced on the Kansas/Colorado border for 25 years. I didn't think KU Health System knew I existed out here, so I really appreciate what I'm doing now. It's a win/win.

Today, over 63 percent of all counties in Kansas are participating in the Care Collaborative.

"This is a body of work that has taken place over the years that is extremely significant," said Peterman. "We have demonstrable results in the reduction of AMI (acute myocardial infarction) in the state of Kansas, and much more. That's because we went out to do something right for patients. The Care Collaborative has had great impact, because it has gotten us connected to other providers in the state. With these leaders, partnerships have been formed that are pretty phenomenal."

LEADERSHIP LESSON:

We leveraged connections nurtured in rural communities from a single project into formal partnerships that enabled us to expand our footprint state-wide. Now even in the remotest regions of the state, there are opportunities for patients to access the resources of a world-class academic medical center. That's a huge benefit, particularly during a major health crisis.

Drawing heavily on those partnerships, KU Health System expanded its footprint to hundreds of locations across the largest population centers: Wichita, Overland Park, Kansas City, and Topeka. To serve rural Kansans, the expansion of campuses to Great Bend, Pawnee Valley, and Hays further ensured patients in those regions have access to high-quality care and the resources of a world-class academic medical center closer to home.

The next advance was compelled by "stay-at-home" orders during the COVID-19 pandemic.

"The need to be accessible to our patients was urgent—including those in rural areas of the state," said Brenda Dykstra, senior vice president and chief strategy officer at TUKHS. "Telehealth became one of our key strategies for serving patients under these circumstances. We had that program standing up within two weeks' time; within 12 weeks, we'd served over 60,000 patients via telehealth."[18]

On-campus specialists were collaborating with off-site physicians to assess patients' issues and create care plans. For patients being referred to specialists, many appointments were managed through a telehealth visit for both initial visits and post-treatment/post-operative follow-ups.

Dykstra noted, "Our telehealth program keeps growing. It's been so helpful in enhancing partnerships across the state and supporting the best patient outcomes."

HOW WE KNOW THAT

Advancing Our Borders: Beyond and Within

We know one of the strongest determinants of lifespan is a person's zip code.[19] That is particularly true in Kansas, a state that has many large underinsured patient populations. Over 34 percent of its counties are designated as "frontier" (those with a population density of less than six per square mile). Providing patients with the most advanced care possible often means bringing that care to them.

One of the strongest determinants of lifespan is a person's zip code.

One of our real advantages is *our* zip code—our location in the center of the country. The expectation of the state legislature is for this health system to "provide patient care and specialized services not widely available elsewhere." This means being innovative, collaborative, and present in the ways we support access to care across the state. And it means sharing what we learn here with healthcare organizations across the country.

Our Care Collaborative is just one of our initiatives to serve the wider community and state. Working side by side with first responders and hospitals across the state, we made significant strides in reducing the short- and longer-term impacts of acute heart attack and acute stroke. Those model practices have already been shared across the country. The collaborative platform, and the shared governance model directing its work, have allowed us to expand beyond those initial diagnoses into other disease and system work, including heart failure and trauma care. The sustainability of this model is replicable across the nation today.

Either through telehealth or on-site presence, our staff and clinicians are supporting access to care where patients live and physicians practice. Our pediatric cystic fibrosis team travels to our outreach clinic in Pittsburg, Kansas, so patients can see the same CF physician, nurse, social worker, dietitian, pharmacist, and respiratory therapist available at the main campus in Kansas City. We have similar programs in many other specialty areas like cardiology, neurology, and cancer.

Our telehealth model provides opportunities for our physicians to collaborate with physicians across the state in the care of specific patients. It also enables direct care to be provided to patients where they live, whether that is right around the corner or hundreds of miles away.

In the backyard of our main campus, we collaborated with our university partners and organizations already providing community healthcare to stand up a federally qualified health center serving the most at-risk zip codes in the county. This work is increasing access and improving the health of our neighbors.

We've also set up "campus care clinics" in several high schools to provide help with teen pregnancy and OB/GYN needs. At our Campus Care Clinic at Topeka High

School, we provided training to staff there and tech support to do telehealth visits during the COVID-19 pandemic. From the comfort of their own homes, teens and families were able to have meaningful interaction with our care providers. The Neonatal Medical Home we created may well be the first of its kind to provide ongoing care to the tiniest of infants after they can go home.

Long before the opioid epidemic, we created and shared the model nationwide for nurse-led pain management teams working side by side with providers and staff to provide therapeutic approaches to reduce patient suffering.

And, in collaboration with our academic partners, we are working to recruit and support talented clinicians. Many have trained here and want to maintain a relationship with an academic medical center as they provide patient care services in communities across the state. We're also promoting healthcare careers by co-facilitating an on-campus science curriculum for high-school juniors and seniors with public school partners.

In a myriad of ways, The University of Kansas Health System is advancing population health and the best of healthcare from our own backyard and beyond our borders…we're not just in Kansas anymore.
—Bob Page

Advancing Leadership

There is a profound connection between extending excellent care out into the community and grooming leadership. The men and women who carry the TUKHS mission outward are carefully selected and trained for this important role.

Adam Meier's career ladder provides a good example of structured leadership development and advancement at KU Health System. After being hired as a unit coordinator, he was promoted within seven months to unit manager. He helped plan, develop, and open Cambridge Tower A in 2017, a new 11-story, $385 million inpatient facility adjacent to the Center for Advanced Heart Care on the health system's main campus.

As part of the clinical team, Meier led a multi-disciplinary endeavor that mapped out all the ways that staff, patients, equipment, medication, and information would flow through the expanded facility. Additionally, during the month leading up to the opening of the new building, Meier's director gave him more opportunities, including leading daily huddles, maintaining a go-live checklist, and working across departments to ensure IT, pharmacy, bio-med, and all related support services were ready to help support the clinical care in Tower A. For Meier, who went on to become director of nursing, ambulatory, and chair of the Nursing Operations Advisory Council, it was an incredible experience.

"Being a part of an amazing team of nurses and leaders who opened this building provided me insight, leadership, and opportunities that are priceless," he said.

Liz Carlton, RN, VP of Quality and Safety, agreed.

"The leadership opportunities abound if you are willing," she said. "I have been provided the opportunity to lead many teams, develop several programs, and stretch beyond my core skill set. I began as a program manager for the trauma program. Shortly thereafter, we added the burn program and the transfer center. In 2008, I was promoted to director of nursing. I kept the programs I had and added quality, safety, and regulatory compliance as well as education and development, Magnet, and infection prevention and control (IPAC).

"In 2015, I was promoted to senior director," Carlton went on. "I've also had the opportunity to develop and/or lead the departments of Nursing Informatics, Youth Sports Medicine, the Center for Concussion Management, the Center for Transplantation, and the Simulation Center." And in 2019, Carlton was promoted to an executive position within the Quality & Safety Dyad.

LEADERSHIP LESSON:

Whenever possible, grow your own and promote from within. Advancing careers from within validates the desired behaviors and increases trust in leadership.

Such opportunities for career advancement abound.

"We love to 'grow our own' and look for leadership potential with every hire we make," Tammy Peterman acknowledged. "I remember getting a call from Beth Clark, one of our former nursing directors. Beth told me she'd just hired a future CNO: Rachel Pepper. After graduating as a member of the first NRP, Rachel's leadership skills became evident and she was promoted to increasingly higher levels of responsibility. Today, she is the CNO of the Kansas City Division, a true example of growing our own. Advancing careers from within validates the behaviors we like to see and shows our employees we're willing to invest in their future."

But the bar is set high, and expectations go with the new territory. Patient and Family-Centered Services Director Rebecca Moburg, RN, remembered her first day as a nurse at KU Hospital.

"It was that great combination of being terrified and excited all at the same time," she recalled. "I walked through the door and I knew the culture. I had made it."

Moburg had worked at other hospitals for 15 years before arriving at what she called "the pinnacle of my career."

"I came here because I was ready and looking for the fast pace," she said. "Where can I learn the most? Where are the sickest patients? Where can I do the most good?"

She managed one of the nursing units for two years before being promoted to an administrative position. Many in her shoes have walked that path.

Tammy Peterman is clear, "We are looking for leadership qualities, but also the right fit for this culture."

HOW WE KNOW THAT

Leadership in a Pandemic

We are dealing with the reality of a pandemic as this book goes to print. Many things we're still learning, but as we came together in the face of COVID-19, some things we already knew. The challenge wasn't providing care—we are more than capable of taking care of the sickest of sick patients here. It was doing everything we could to keep our patients and employees safe, and to provide leadership that would inspire confidence and calm.

Communication is the key—both internally and externally. We do what we have long prepared to do—we activate our incident command and surge plans, review and adapt emergency management plans with all our service lines and supply chains, and ramp up technology and telemedicine so we can diagnose and treat more patients remotely.

Through initiatives like our "Take-10" news-style updates and our 24/7 intranet info-feed, we focus our internal communications on proactive direction to our physicians and staff. And we use a wide variety of platforms to reach our patients and our community (see Chapter 9), as well as delivering accurate information to the media.

We also provide leadership within the broader healthcare community. When hospitals in this area were getting their first confirmed patients, Bob and I were exchanging texts with the other CEOs to try to reach some consensus on issues we're all experiencing. At times like this, it's not about competition—it's about cooperation. Everyone looks to our health system for leadership, so we take that responsibility seriously.

LEADERSHIP LESSON:

At times like this, it's not about competition—it's about cooperation.

Since our Medical News Network has an in-house studio, we immediately made it available to state and local officials, including U.S. Senator for Kansas

Jerry Moran and Dr. Lee Norman, secretary of the Kansas Department of Health and Environment, to broadcast a series of news conferences with our medical experts. We also began airing targeted "bench-to-bedside" segments and kept a steady stream of news flowing about the developing aspects of this pandemic. All of that was reinforced on our general website and via internal communications, so staff was getting consistent updates on the issues within our health system.

Keeping people in the know is so important, because fear is mostly about the unknown. People need a stabilizing force of calm; they need to see leadership in that mode. Our circular communication process was already in place, so people were just doing even more of that: checking in with you—asking how your family is doing, how you're feeling. That support helps us all cope.

LEADERSHIP LESSON:

It's not about titles; it's about who has the best idea…and that could be a different person the next day. Your culture has to support that kind of collaboration. You'll need it in a time of crisis.

Our collaborative culture was demonstrated in so many ways. If you were looking in on a command center huddle, you couldn't tell what anybody's title was—it's about who has the best idea, and that could be a different person the next day. I thought many times how important it's been for us to hire not just for skill, but for will. This collaborative, leadership-at-all-levels culture that puts patients first was already in place, so the agility we needed was there in a time of crisis.
—Tammy Peterman

The right fit is a combination of cultural and professional competence, and that special knowing "how to connect—which is what patients and family members need when they are in crisis," Moburg asserts. "Yes, patients need great, high-quality care. They need infection prevention and skilled surgeons and everything else, but patients also need us to connect with them—that creates the best patient experience and helps produce the best outcomes."

LEADERSHIP LESSON:

Patients need us to connect with them—not just as doctors and nurses, but as human beings. That makes the best experience and helps produce the best outcomes.

CHAPTER NINE

Celebrate It

Celebrate what you've accomplished,
but raise the bar a little higher each time you succeed.
—Mia Hamm

Small slips of paper are folded into the cracks of the limestone block wall in Bell Sanctuary at The University of Kansas Health System, each with a handwritten message. The first thing the young woman in the chemo scarf does when she enters the chapel just inside the main foyer is write her note and add it to the others there: *Last week, the nurses sang* We Will Rock You—*I love them! Today, we're celebrating because I'm in the final week of treatment. And I'm going to be okay.*

Celebrations at KU Health System come in many different forms. From a deeply personal moment at the prayer wall or in a patient's room, to the time set aside in each department to recognize an employee's professional achievement, each observance had its beginning as a story. And in a culture of affirmation, those stories get shared organically and curated purposefully.

Encouraging stories and sharing them both informally and formally produces a ready source of exemplars.

Celebrating those shining moments with official recognition creates the mechanism and motivation for cultural definition, positivity, and sustainability.

Stories are the cultural currency of this health system.

The importance of celebrating the good things "is not only because it's good for the spirit, it's good for the body—including the corporate body," Chief Culture Officer Terry Rusconi points out. "We know positivity can improve people's outlook, support resilience, and enable each individual to contribute their talents to the fullest. So we've elevated it within our culture as an organization. Celebrating achievements by sharing our stories is the cultural currency of this health system."

LEADERSHIP LESSON:

The importance of celebrating the good things is not only because it's good for the spirit, it's good for the body—including the corporate body. Positivity can improve people's outlook, support resilience, and enable each individual to contribute their talents to the fullest, so we've elevated the importance of celebration within our culture as an organization.

The Cultural Currency

Sharing stories and celebrating intentionally began with the transformation of the hospital back in 1998.

"We started doing that in our management team meetings," recalled Jon Jackson, who retired as KU Health System Senior VP in 2017. "When Bob Page became chief operating officer, he did a lot of it. Tammy Peterman did it a lot, too. We started telling stories about patients we had successfully interacted with, and things that we were getting compliments on."

Here's what I see when I think about the dedication of the people who work here: One of the valets who works at our oncology clinic...the day he had a giant tool box, and was fixing a patient's loose license plate while she was getting her radiation treatments. That's what it looks like.
—Gigi Siers, MS, RN, NE-BC

The feel-good aspect was validating, but the strategy came to serve another purpose as well. Stories are positive reinforcement of cultural values aligning thousands of individual employees to a consistent organizational vision.

LEADERSHIP LESSON:

Stories are positive reinforcement of cultural values aligning thousands of individual employees to a consistent organizational vision.

Validating good work unites everyone in a sense of pride and community. When self-esteem aligns to group-esteem, the culture is strengthened.

"It's incredibly important to share our stories," says Kayla Northrop, RN. "We use stories to draw new people in and help them feel a part of an ongoing story—so they know they're continuing the story of this hospital."

When self-esteem aligns to group-esteem, this strengthens cultural assimilation.

The Parable of the Flood

When stories of individual impact are pervasive in the culture, it has an empowering, collective effect. The efficacy of each person on the team and the team as a whole are heightened, so even significant problems are easier to solve—like a big flood in the foyer.

It happened about 7:00 a.m. on October 30, 2019, when many of our teams were beginning a new shift. A central hot water line burst above our second-floor clinical lab. Water spewed across the floor, down through the ceiling of the floor below, streaming over the walls of the main entrance. Many patients had just begun to arrive for their scheduled procedures. This wasn't a small leak; it was a flood—a big mess with significant fall-risk for patients and staff, and risk of permanent damage to essential patient care equipment.

Here's what was so amazing: Everyone already knew what to do—even though this particular problem had never occurred before.

It took a couple of hours to fix the pipe, but no one shut down waiting for someone up the chain of command to advise next steps…no instructions from on-high, no frustrating delays to action. There was no debate, no crisis of leadership, and there were "no tears." Instead, the question asked was the only one that mattered: *What can we do right now for our patients?*

In one of the areas of biggest impact, Admitting and the Pre-Anesthesia Clinic (PAC), everybody just dove in. Admitting transferred its operations into the lobby of the Center for Advanced Heart Care, and PAC moved temporarily to the fourth floor of the Medical Pavilion. By that afternoon, systems were back online and up to speed. Although it required a few more days to complete necessary physical repairs, direct patient-care services didn't miss a beat.[1]
—Liz Carlton, Vice President of Quality & Safety

At every orientation, Bob Page invites new employees to be part of the unfolding story of this health system. Stories are shared throughout the orientation process. They establish the true north of expectations while encouraging and inspiring equally powerful stories from those individuals joining the TUKHS team.

"We want everyone here to recognize and own their part in creating our story," Page said.

New Employee Orientation: A Compass Story

Pam is an exceptional employee who goes above and beyond for our patients. It's not uncommon for her to walk up to the front lobby to give patients a hug or share a tear. She is quick to assure patients that they're in good hands, easing their anxiety. Her dedication really showed with a new patient referral. This young man suffered from agoraphobia—and he was an hour away! She guided him to try making small trips toward our office, going a little farther each day. It took two to three months for the patient to gain the courage to make it the full distance, but Pam kept in touch with him the entire time, cheering him on. She's a wonderful patient advocate and a joy to work with.

—Jennifer Hill, Former Office Supervisor, Sarcoma Center

From huddles in each unit to a daily intranet newsfeed system-wide, telling stories keeps it real and works against routinization. It distinguishes the extraordinary while grounding the value system.

Tammy Peterman also believes "it keeps things relevant and personal. We want everyone to feel that sense of personal connection and belonging that promotes loyalty and trust."

Compassionate Care

At her funeral, her husband described the sun coming through the windows and the five dark weeks of losing his wife all of a sudden becoming brighter when these "two angels" came into the room.

These two angels were our nurses who created a "spa day" to help his wife leave the hospital with dignity. A year after she passed, he shared the story in a ceremony to recognize these nurses for the "magical, unbelievable time" they created for his wife to feel and look as beautiful as possible for herself and her family as she went home to die.

He announced an endowment to go on forever. Annually, the recipient will receive a check for $1,000 to spend at a spa or a weekend away—whatever would give that nurse the feeling his wife and family knew, thanks to such compassionate care.
—Chris Ruder, RN, COO

Narrative Structure

Messages in the limestone prayer wall in Bell Sanctuary are just one of many ways story-sharing is literally structured into the health system and its culture. Numerous mechanisms are in place system-wide to capture uplifting accounts that emphasize the "good news" that happens every day at TUKHS. For example:

- Feel-good human interest stories and good news posted on the website, www.KansasHealthSystem.com
- A 24/7 intranet where staff going above and beyond are profiled
- TUKHS Annual Report
- Inspiring news of medical trials, treatment successes, and cutting-edge techniques shared on the Medical News Network
- Social media platforms including Facebook, Instagram, Twitter @KUHospital, and a YouTube channel
- Blog-style stories that emphasize wellness and recovery on the website
- *Good Medicine*, a hard-copy news magazine about patients, care providers, donors, and events
- E-newsletters focusing on a variety of topics:
    - *BeWell Connection* features healthy recipes and lifestyle tips
    - *Pulse* offers heart-healthy news
    - *Catalyst* provides the latest news in research and treatment plus inspirational stories for cancer patients
    - *Good Medicine Connection* is full of real patient stories and upcoming events of interest to the community
- Take-10, a daily internal broadcast begun in March 2020 featuring Bob Page and Tammy Peterman, along with topic experts and staffers sharing COVID-19 and other updates
- Event sponsorships:

- American Heart Association Heart Walk®
- Race for the Cure
- United Way
- The Stroke Walk

- HERO—this Health System Employees Reaching Out initiative hosts many volunteer programs during the year, from teaching youngsters about bicycle safety to scraping paint from elderly neighbors' homes during "Christmas in October"
- Turning Point, a center to meet, listen, share, learn, and encourage with classes and resiliency training for patients

Sharing What She Learned: "I would never take back having had cancer."

In August 2013, active mom Emily Dumler was surprised to discover blood in her stool. Her doctor advised her to go directly to a nearby emergency room, so she told her three young children and husband she'd be back in an hour or so. "Instead, I was admitted to the hospital, where I stayed for 43 days," Dumler said.

Emily, then 32, had non-Hodgkin lymphoma. After treatment at another hospital and MD Anderson Cancer Center, she eventually came to The University of Kansas Cancer Center.

"I was told that my only chance at a cure was CAR T-cell immunotherapy," Emily said. While some CAR T-cell therapies have become FDA-approved to treat certain types of cancers, its effects were unknown at the time. Still, she signed up for the trial.

Emily was only the third patient in the world to receive CAR T-cell immunotherapy. "We just didn't know what would happen," Emily said. And many side effects that could occur, did occur. During her infusion, a sinus problem intensified, and her IV was temporarily stopped so she could receive an antihistamine. Later, she experienced flu-like symptoms followed by neurological toxicity.

"They watched for that very, very closely," she says. "They did cognitive exams several times a day, asking questions that seemed so silly—like did I know my name, and could I name a shape—until I couldn't answer them. I ended up losing my cognitive function and my memory for about 24 to 36 hours. Fortunately, medications reversed all those side effects in time."

Today, Emily is healthy and strong. She returned to employment outside the home and enjoys attending her children's many sporting events with her husband. She still visits her care team once or twice a year, but believes the cancer is gone. Her experience has brought a significant new perspective.

Despite the challenges and the low points she and her family experienced, Emily wouldn't change her journey.

"It may be easier for me to say because of where I'm sitting today, but I would never take back having had cancer," she says. "I am a different person for it, and for the better. I learned so much about myself and what is truly important in life. And I signed up for the trial for myself, to save my own life, but there is so much that is coming from these efforts, so much for the cancer community to gain. It is amazing to be some part of that, and I feel truly blessed."

Emily's good news was celebrated at KU Health System across internal and external platforms. In February 2018, Emily and her doctor, Joseph McGuirk, DO, director of hematologic malignancies and cellular therapeutics at KU Cancer Center, shared their story on "Medical Mysteries and Miracles" with *Megyn Kelly Today.*[2]

Intentional Focus on the Good

Hospitals are often fraught with stress and anxiety. The intentional pursuit of good news is crucial and healing. At KU Health System, inspirational stories form an interconnected narrative that both supports and encourages transcendent efforts.

Drawings and thank-you cards from the community make it to me. One was a three-page poem from a prisoner at Lansing Correctional Facility whom we treated for COVID-19. He took the time to share his appreciation with this extraordinary gesture. I could have just shared it with the Emergency Department and Unit 61, but instead, I submitted it for a DAISY Team Award for an interdisciplinary, nurse-led COVID-19 team. The story was also shared on the website in our "24/7" staff news feature.

This is our mindset: to not just appreciate what's happening here, but to look for ways to share and celebrate these amazing stories as broadly as possible.
—Gigi Siers

"We want to make sure we're taking every opportunity to spotlight and celebrate the amazing things going on here," Bob Page said. "Our people are bringing help and hope to patients facing some of the worst days of their lives. One of the reasons Tammy and I like to join rounds is to hear those stories firsthand so we can share them widely."

LEADERSHIP LESSON:

Hospital environments are often fraught with stress and anxiety. The intentional pursuit of good news is crucial. Uplifting stories form an interconnected narrative that both supports and encourages transcendent efforts.

When major events or just water-cooler conversations are infused with intention, "You raise the emotional waters around you," write *Thriving in Healthcare* coauthors Wayne M. Sotile, PhD, and Gary R. Simonds, MD, MHCDS.[3] "As you give off your 'positive waves,' others begin to synchronize and resonate. Soon, a 'ripples in the pond' effect may take place. You develop a network of positive and engaged contacts. This all helps to offset the negative impact of the depressing and hostile miasma that sometimes fills healthcare environments."

LEADERSHIP LESSON:

Create mechanisms for finding and sharing stories.

Actively Capturing Stories from the Daily Provision of Care

One of the most important lessons learned early in the organization's transformation was the importance of creating structures so stories could be captured and shared across the health system. Without intentional structures, great stories can be missed and opportunities to recognize and inspire passed by. Here are some mechanisms the organization uses:

- Encourage patients to fill out a feedback card with any good thoughts for a staff member
- Direct managers to note stories they hear from patients/families during rounds
- Invite staff to share stories of what they observed/heard about another staff member
- Listen to the stories new employees tell about why they want to work here
- Build time into regular meetings for sharing stories
- Start huddles with a positive story
- Ensure stories are a part of key external events so the community understands the values driving the organization

Deploying a Good Story

Daran was a high school senior who'd already enlisted in the Marine's delayed-entry program. He couldn't wait to get to basic training after graduation, but began having headaches and double vision. He was diagnosed with a very serious brain tumor—the kind with about a 2 percent chance for survival.

The first thing I noticed as I walked onto the ICU was a Marine in full dress uniform guarding the entrance to Daran's room. The Marines remained at that post out of respect for Daran, this boy who would never get the chance to join the Marines. That's an image none of us will ever forget. There wasn't a dry eye on the unit.

I got to know Daran's family well. I remember his dad asking Dr. Taylor, Daran's oncologist, about his son's odds of survival. Dr. Taylor replied, "I didn't come here to talk with you about his odds of survival; I came here to talk to you about how we are going to cure him."

It was just about that time that I myself began experiencing debilitating headaches. About one month into that, I had a CT scan that showed something. A quick MRI confirmed it: I had a walnut-sized cyst that was stretching my optic nerve.

Dr. Chamoun, my neurosurgeon, told me I'd need a full craniotomy to remove it. The only words I could speak were, "I am so freaked out that I can't hear you right now."

So I had to give Daran the news that, like him, I was going to have a craniotomy. His first words were, "I will be there for you, Aunt Gigi."

After my surgery, each and every time I woke up in my hospital room, Daran and his dad were there to greet me. I was able to go home after four days, but I couldn't drive. Two weeks out of my craniotomy, I got a text from Daran reminding me of a promise I'd made, "It's my last day of chemo, so now you can show me the best view of Kansas City."

It was a Sunday and I wasn't allowed to drive yet, but a promise is a promise. A friend took me to the hospital, and I met Daran in his room on the oncology floor and escorted him to the secret destination: the TUKHS helipad!

I had a swift recovery and was back to work in three weeks. One of the things that I do at The University of Kansas Health System is teach customer service to new employees. It occurred to me that Daran could fill some of his long hours during radiation treatments and convalescence by coming to class and sharing his perspective as a patient with my classes. It was an immediate hit, and we made it an official part of the training curriculum.

Then and now, Daran always says the one thing every patient needs is a smile. When someone is really sick, there aren't a lot of smiles amongst family and friends. That smile and easy-going banter with staff were often the high point of his day. Daran shares that with new employees. That's pretty insightful for an 18-year-old kid, right?

Daran also encourages new employees to ask patients what they did before they were sick, and what they are going to do once they're well again. Hearing his story is powerful; usually, there's not a dry eye in the house. The message resonates with everyone.

Since he seemed to enjoy talking to new staff, I invited him to speak to our "Nurse Academy," a program for prospective nurses who are still in high school. Daran liked sharing his experience as a patient. "Everyone makes a difference in this hospital," he'd say. "You don't have to be a doctor or a nurse or a patient care assistant. Everyone—from the people who deliver food or clean the rooms—made a difference for me when they came in with a smile."

Despite missing most of his senior year during treatment, Daran still managed to graduate with his class. But an even bigger highlight was the trip he made to Washington, DC, as a special guest of the commandant and sergeant major of the United States Marine Corps. Thanks to the Dream Factory, the Wankums were invited to the Marine Corps War Memorial. In a special ceremony that included an eight-man rifle volley, Daran was designated an honorary Marine. He is only the 22nd individual to have ever received this honor in the history of the Corps.

We celebrate that with him, and share his story—which is also our story—with our new employees at orientation.[4]

—Gigi Siers

Motivation Contagion

Celebrating KU Health System culture in action is standard operating procedure without being routine. It's still special—and it works, although it took some time to figure out how it worked best.

"In the early days, the low morale was palpable...we had a lot of work to do just to build trust in leadership. We wanted staff to see our faces and know we were there for them—even at 2:00 in the morning. We'd literally show up and take the time to talk with folks working the night shift," Bob Page recalled.

"At that time, our patient satisfaction ranking was so low, we were trying everything we could think of to even reach the 50th percentile," Page explained. "Tammy and I asked (then-CEO) Irene Thompson if we could give everybody $50 to celebrate if we reached that goal. We got that approved, but we didn't reach the 50th percentile that year and no one received $50. That's when we began to realize, in our culture, a financial reward wasn't the motivation to move the dial," he added.

If you wait for people to go above and beyond, you'll never get to the reward and recognition they need to be inspired to go above and beyond.[5]
—Quint Studer

Of the various strategies employed to improve performance in those days, it was a banner that finally got the desired response. It read *OUR PATIENTS AND VISITORS SAID YOU WERE THE BEST! THANK YOU!*

Peterman said, "Every Friday, Bob and I personally delivered this big banner ceremoniously to the unit that got the best patient satisfaction survey results for the week. We made a very big deal out of it. Word got around. The next week, we'd move the banner to the next unit with the highest performance. Ultimately, we purchased dozens of banners to recognize units with patient satisfaction at the 90th percentile or higher."

Every week, the pride of ownership sparked a friendly competition and engaged more and more units in the performance improvement process.

HOW WE KNOW THAT

Accountability and Celebration: Two Sides of the Same Coin

As an executive, trying to celebrate going from the 5th percentile on patient satisfaction to the 10th percentile was hard. I was thinking, *Really?* But it was incredibly important for us to do that. I remember telling Irene I wasn't impressed by the places that had self-proclaimed quality and internal awards. I said, "Let's not do that." But she told me, "Bob, it's really important for this organization to get anything." Those days taught me a lot about how we need to celebrate every step along the way to our goal.

LEADERSHIP LESSON:

We started from such a low point of performance, it felt overwhelming. But we learned it's really important to celebrate every small step along the way to our goal.

At one point, Tammy and I took a really ratty old cart and painted it bright colors and then we stocked it with treats. We would take candy bars and all kinds of other stuff—nothing healthy. Then we would go shift-by-shift, unit-by-unit, and department-by-department as an executive team. We would go out with that cart just to thank people for their work…for every effort to go the extra mile. A Snickers bar at 11:00 at night is kind of like a piece of gold. The staff was amazed that executives were in the house at that time of night for no reason other than to show them some appreciation.

So it was real simple stuff because we didn't have a lot of money to do big stuff. But we engaged in this directly as executive leaders—we didn't delegate it to other people. We actually got out there and got to know our staff so we could recognize and reward them appropriately.

LEADERSHIP LESSON:

It was real simple stuff because we didn't have a lot of money to do big stuff. But we engaged in this directly as executive leaders—we didn't delegate it to other people.

It wasn't just an "attaboy" thing—we also focused on accountability. Celebrating current performance without holding people accountable to advance performance could result in the ultimate goal remaining out of reach.

When Tammy was chief nurse and I was COO, we would block four hours every Friday, and the manager of any unit that had patient satisfaction below the threshold would come down and spend 15 minutes with us going over the surveys from their unit. We'd walk them through the numbers and listen to their thoughts on why patient satisfaction was low. We'd ask questions and discuss solutions. I could see the progress when these meetings went from taking up the whole morning to taking up half of the morning...and then only one-third of the morning. The units were starting to get over that threshold. They knew it was important to this organization, and they were going to be held accountable for it.

Then we started to build an incentive system where we would compensate leaders for accomplishing organizational goals—not just their individual goals—and we built recognition into that process.

Today, we view patient satisfaction as everyone's job. It's not just a unit goal; it's an executive goal—even the people in accounting are held to the same expectation as clinical people for patient satisfaction.

Everyone here impacts the patient experience in one way or another, whether you're touching a patient clinically or not. All of us are accountable. Motivating that behavior includes rewarding and celebrating it.
—Bob Page

LEADERSHIP LESSON:

We found monetary rewards weren't the strongest incentive. In a people-first culture, having the respect of peers is a much bigger motivation.

Consistent with what American philosopher William James posited—that the deepest principle in human nature is the craving to be appreciated—Page and Peterman learned that money was not the incentive that worked best in this culture.

"It's having the respect of your peers and having your best efforts recognized and appreciated," Peterman said. "It's knowing you helped that patient get better, or that family member feel supported. Those things really validated and motivated our staff. And they still do."

Bob and Tammy are present, even on weekends. That cannot be undervalued in terms of a leader's commitment to an organization. Their presence has been critical, to discuss a course correction during a difficult situation or to celebrate.
—Jeff Wright, VP of Cancer Services

The Celebration Cycle

Celebration isn't about braggadocio; it's about refreshing the frame of reference that keeps everyone connected to performance goals.

Nurse-Nominated Doctor Awards

The first thing I noticed about Dr. Bayrak is that she is team-centered. She was immediately willing to help do things that were not "her job" in order to facilitate an efficient, safe, and healing operating room (like getting warm blankets, opening items for the scrub, answering the phone, etc.). I am a circulating nurse in Cambridge OR, and actions like these speak louder than words. Dr. Bayrak is always willing to help by going above and beyond expectations. She is compassionate on calls that other people

may find annoying or a waste of their time (it sometimes is), but she is always patient with the people on the other end of the line asking the questions. She has a fantastic memory when it comes to her patients; it shows how much she genuinely cares. Dr. Bayrak is walking quality. She looks to improve every time I work with her. If everyone worked as hard as she does, the world would be a better place. It's obvious that Dr. Bayrak makes sure she is informed, prepared, and knowledgeable about what the plans are for the patient before she ever steps foot in the OR. I have genuine confidence when I tell my patients that they are going to receive phenomenal care when Dr. Sinehan Bayrak is the resident in the OR.
—Jessica Farmer, RN

Reflecting on his experience in working with hospitals across the country, Chris Drummond with Huron Consulting Group noted, "Hospitals and their executives are hard on themselves and commonly fail at celebrating and communicating their wins and improvements. It's important to their staff, patients, communities, and other stakeholders that this performance data be widely shared and celebrated."

Celebration isn't about braggadocio; it's about refreshing the frame of reference that keeps everyone connected to performance goals.

Good deeds and good data go hand in hand, so stories and performance statistics are channeled through a celebration cycle.

Celebration Cycle Components

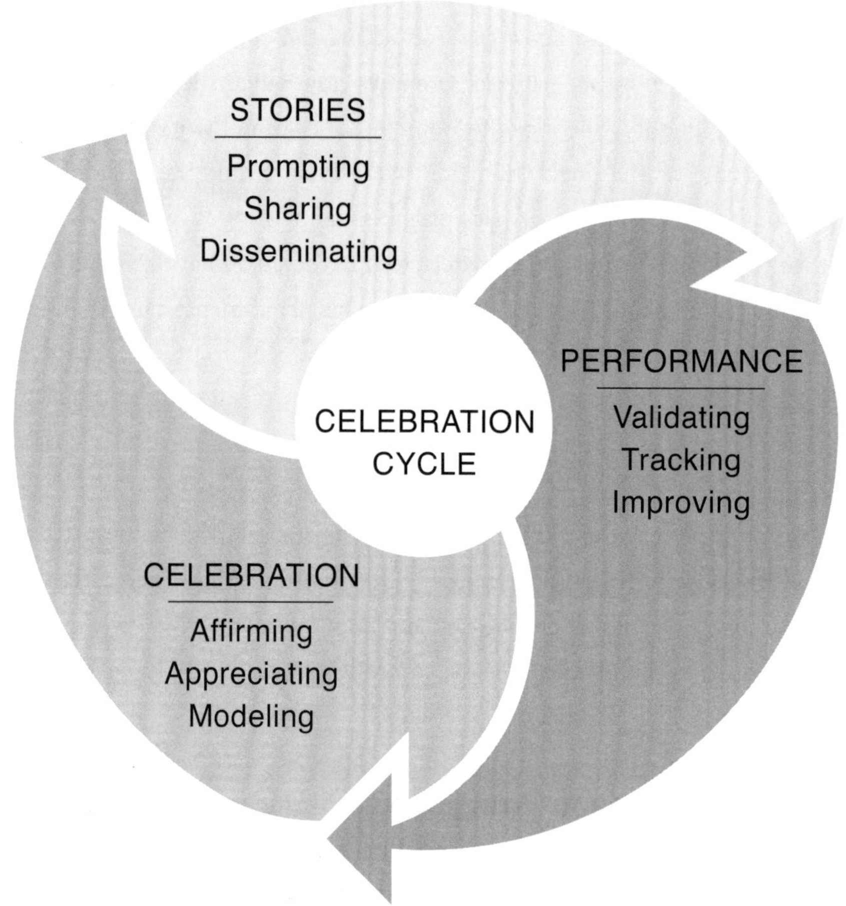

HOW WE KNOW THAT

Celebration as Strategy

When it comes to celebrating achievements, what happens on the unit doesn't stay on the unit! We want that good news to travel to other departments, management, executive leadership, and even to patients and out to the community. Sometimes a team from a unit will be invited to come share their story with our board of directors or at our local, regional, and national professional meetings.

Even small stories can get special recognition, because many units create their own ways to highlight good news. Awards or commendations are often created as packaging for that group's particular brand of greatness, and we encourage that.

The "Good Catch" award is just one example. In our Kansas City Division, anyone "caught" in the act of preventing harm to a patient can be nominated for this recognition. By actually celebrating that, we're making a strong statement to our employees that they're empowered to do the right thing. This can keep things from getting swept under the rug because everyone's afraid to take the blame.

In addition to Good Catch, we have a long list of awards we've either created or take part in. Many have been established in honor of a patient we've treated, including:

- 19 Donor-Supported Awards
- IPAC (Infection Prevention and Control) Award
- Excellence in Caring Award
- Nursing Excellence Awards
- Outstanding Resident Award
- Attending Physician Awards
- March of Dimes Nurse of the Year Awards
- DAISY Awards
    - For Extraordinary Nursing
    - DAISY Leader
    - DAISY in Training
    - DAISY Team
    - DAISY Champion

Nursing has been particularly good at the celebration cycle. We take time each year to formally recognize every nurse who maintains professional certification. And we encourage staff to seek out opportunities to nominate their peers or units for awards whether internal or from an outside source. We're proud when we're recognized, but never satisfied. Recognition is a way of saying, *Look, here's where the bar is set…what can we do to clear it?*
—Tammy Peterman

Hall of Fame

When Bob Page came up with the idea for a "Hall of Fame" at The University of Kansas Health System, he was feeling that the "crowd swell doesn't just happen in sports; it happens in healthcare, too."

The feeling of exuberance that rises out of a collective pride in achievement was the genesis of his idea.

"We have so much to be proud of here—so many really stellar individuals who have been part of writing and telling our story," said Page. "I really wanted to create an opportunity to thank them and our partner organizations for the vital role they've played in our efforts to deliver world-class care to patients most in need. We want them to know their leadership, philanthropy, and advocacy will leave a lasting impact."

Three categories of awards are given during the annual induction ceremony:

- The Legacy
- The Catalyst
- The Partner in Excellence

The Hall of Fame event brings health system and medical staff leadership together with the wider community of stakeholders to celebrate what they've achieved through shared commitment and collaboration. The dinner event is intentionally not a fundraiser; it's a celebration of people and partners who have been joined in this endeavor.

Story Ambassadors

"Talking story" is not just an internal process. Hall of Fame honoree Charles Sunderland has been on the TUKHS Board of Directors for over 18 years—many of them as chair of the quality committee. Sunderland looks for opportunities to tout KU Health System. "I never hesitate to recommend KU Health System to anybody interested in improving their health. I bring up the quality of care, the AMC concept, the teams of doctors you can access with so many specialists. It's pretty easy to be a cheerleader for the hospital when I see the good work that's happening here."

Choose to Celebrate

Whether high five, group hug, or highest honors—celebration as ritual is a way to reinforce the organizational vision. When built into the culture, it becomes a way to relentlessly but creatively communicate the practical applications of that vision.

"Every day there's something to celebrate when you're using positivity for climate control," Tammy Peterman explained. "As leaders, we can adjust attitudes across our entire organization by choosing to celebrate what's going well."

LEADERSHIP LESSON:

Two of the most important reasons to "Celebrate It" are 1) to relentlessly but creatively communicate and reinforce your vision; and 2) to use positivity as organizational climate control.

Bob and Tammy,

I am a new employee at your organization. During orientation, current employees spoke about how everyone has a story and something that brought them here. This is my third week here, and I wanted to share my story with you.

I graduated from The University of Kansas School of Nursing in 2009. My passion was pediatrics, and I spent the next eight years working with critically ill pediatric patients. I loved my job and I never imagined leaving.

Then August 2, 2017, arrived.

Only 25 days earlier, I'd given birth to a beautiful baby girl. She wasn't even a month old when I found myself sitting in a hematologist's office at another local hospital hearing someone tell me I had leukemia. I needed to be admitted to the hospital within the next 24 hours to begin treatment and would be inpatient for the next five to six weeks. My first thought was my children. *How do I leave my new baby and four-year-old son?*

How is my husband going to take care of them and continue working? Who will help care for my family if I die? These questions were racing through my mind.

The hematologist and a well-respected oncologist laid out the treatment plan. They said they would give me until the next day to be admitted. I liked and respected these doctors, but honestly, when I heard the word "cancer," only one hospital came to mind: The University of Kansas Health System.

My mother was with me, but she had stepped out of that appointment to call her long-time friend, Liz Carlton, a nurse at TUKHS. Liz started the ball rolling, and within a few hours, I received a phone call from one of your physicians, Dr. Lin. She explained my type of cancer and the rationale to start treatment that night instead of waiting for a consultation appointment the next day. This doctor was also a mother. She understood and empathized with me about leaving my children. That phone call meant so much.

When I hung up, I packed my bag, kissed my children goodbye, and my husband drove me to your hospital. I was in a room on Unit 41 by 9:30 that night. Another physician on the team met me in my room and explained everything again and answered my questions. The PICC line was placed and treatment started that very night.

Exactly two weeks later on August 16, I was discharged. In those two weeks, every person I encountered measured up to the standards that were discussed during orientation. My nurses and care assistants were phenomenal! Every single one of them went above and beyond to make sure that I understood my plan of care and that I was as comfortable as I could be living in a hospital. Since children weren't allowed on Unit 41, they arranged for me to move to a larger room that could accommodate my family on Unit 42 within a few days of my admission. Angie, the charge nurse, even obtained a crib so we could put my daughter down when she visited.

Everyone was accommodating on what time they drew labs and got vitals to allow me time with my family without impacting my care. They held my hand while I cried during a painful bone marrow aspiration. They did so much more than their job requires.

Bob and Tammy, it's important for you to see your employees and your hospital as your patients see it. The employees at TUKHS are the best—they took the worst days of my life and made them better. They made my new "normal" an okay way to live for a while. And now you all have given me a chance to get back to doing what I love: being a nurse. It's in a completely different way from how I ever dreamed, but I'm so excited about it!

Thank you for taking such good care of me as a patient and thank you for giving me this opportunity as an employee.[6]
—Katy Edwards, BSN, RN

CHAPTER TEN

Sustain It

Sustainability takes forever. And that's the point.
—William McDonough

In many ways, the abandoned 220,000-square-foot building in downtown Kansas City, Kansas, mirrored another dilemma facing the community: How do we tend to the growing population going without mental health treatment?

It was a big, expensive, complicated problem that no one seemed to want to take on—until The University of Kansas Health System did. The solution developed by TUKHS met the challenge "at a time when many other organizations were reducing or eliminating these services," Tammy Peterman said. "We had to look at the issues right in front of our eyes."

In 2019, KU Health System reopened the doors of that same building. It was now revitalized as the health system's state-of-the-art center for adult mental and behavioral health on its newly named Strawberry Hill Campus.

"This is truly an amazing transformation of an empty office building into a vibrant place for care," said Chris Ruder, RN, COO of the health system's Kansas City Division.

Resurrecting a vacant building in an historic neighborhood is an operational challenge; addressing the issues of mental illness across the community is a fundamental obligation. "Mental illness isn't a sexy problem," Bob Page acknowledged, "but it is a crisis. Population health is our concern. More is, and should be, expected of you when your performance has earned you recognition as a local and national leader. Your expertise, resources, and talent should be directed to take on issues you have not been able to previously address. We took it on at this level because this is a vast, unmet need…that's what we do."

> Helping people is what we should be doing. [TUKHS] occupied a very large vacant building with the sole purpose of handling cases not normally managed by other health systems. It is amazing what has happened in the past 20 years. I predict The University of Kansas Health System will eventually be the number-one health system in the United States.
> —William H. Dunn, Sr., Chairman Emeritus of JE Dunn Construction

Proactivity like this has characterized KU Health System's approach since its transformation began in 1998. Buying the empty building on "Strawberry Hill" in the heart of the city and dedicating it to an underserved population was not only an opportunity, but a necessity. It made a difference to the community on many levels.

Continuous improvement becomes the sustainability model.

"We're always looking for ways to better serve the people who need us. It's about expanding and improving how we do this work," Peterman said. "Not in 'flavor-of-the-month' fashion, but in ways that embody the health system's culture."

Former Board Chair Bob Honse said, "Not only are they always trying to improve, but they are also trying to get better, not necessarily to get bigger. Growth is good if it's good growth."

"We work hard to maintain what we've built," Bob Page explained. "But also to sustain it. It's important to make a distinction between 'maintain' and 'sustain.' You can *maintain* things like equipment or facilities, but you *sustain* a culture—that's a living, improving, ever-expanding organism. Its sustainability is anything but static."

"If you're doing this right, continuous improvement itself becomes the sustainability model that provides that energy and reinforcement," he concluded.

LEADERSHIP LESSON:
Sustainability is anything but static. If you're doing this right, continuous improvement itself becomes the sustainability model.

A Sustainability Model

Survival was the immediate goal when The University of Kansas Hospital became independent from the state system in 1998. With only 30 days of cash in its coffers, revenue was a priority—but not the singular goal. Infrastructuring a values-based organization and providing the best patient care from a staff empowered to do so were the priorities.

"We had a vision of the big picture, and it wasn't driven by profit," Page stated. The hospital was at rock-bottom in those days, in terms of patient satisfaction and other measures. Page knew, "We had to improve to survive.

"So we set our sights on doing that as well as it could possibly be done," he continued. "We were—and still are—committed to that goal."

To create a sustainable process for that, maintenance and improvement were seen as inseparable.[1] The heuristic was quality plus service plus people equaled growth and sustainability: the Five-Star Guiding Formula (see Chapter 2).

That formula has never changed, but the process it directs is anything but fixed.

"If we're always asking better questions, if we're constantly questioning our assumptions every step of the way, then all our initiatives have this in common: improvement," reflected Chief Culture Officer Terry Rusconi. "What we've learned is if we're always improving, we're simultaneously creating sustainability."

If we're always improving, we're simultaneously creating sustainability.

Persistence and a Plan

Sustainability presents particular challenges to "academic health systems [that] have very little room for error since they face unique business disadvantages in the marketplace, including a less favorable payer mix and a traditionally higher overhead due to their academic mission."[2]

Page and Peterman knew survival hinged on the success of the guiding formula. Strategic initiatives that addressed each of the five pillars were developed—all with advancement in mind. As former KUMC Chair of Internal Medicine Susan Pingleton, MD, saw it, they "kept the momentum going by continually challenging themselves."

Acquisition of outpatient services, the development of service lines, and major capital improvements on campus were constantly in the works.

"I would characterize their approach as never sitting still," Pingleton said. "Never saying, *Okay, we're done. We are going to take a three-month break here.* There has always been something that's next."[3]

Over the transformative years since 1998, persistence and a plan produced major milestones for TUKHS.

Strategic Milestones of Sustained Progress

	Foundational
1998	University of Kansas Public Authority established
2000	Regained management of the Cancer Center Expanded cardiovascular services with addition of Mid-America Cardiology & Mid-America Thoracic and Cardiovascular Surgeons
2007	Began initial phase of creating an integrated electronic medical record

2014	Health system commitment to Lean methodology Launched Medical News Network™ (MNN)
2016	"One Health System" announced with inception of clinical integration
2020	Live COVID-19 interactive "media update" is broadcast Monday-Friday from Medical News Network—first locally, then restreamed nationally

	Service/People/Quality
1999-2000	Focus on service recognized by improving patient satisfaction
2000	First certified as ACS Level I Trauma Center
2004	First annual nursing meeting
2006	First designated as a Magnet hospital (redesignated in '11 and '16)
2007	First recognized on *U.S. News & World Report's* Best Hospitals List
2008	First achieved 90th percentile ranking in patient satisfaction[4]
2009	Ranked #2 among comprehensive academic medical centers by University HealthSystem Consortium
2009	Nurse Residency Program became one of the first to be accredited by Commission on Collegiate Nursing Education
2012	The University of Kansas Cancer Center receives first National Cancer Institute (NCI) designation
2013	Received the first PRISM Award for medical-surgical nursing units
2017	Health system receives the first Joint Commission Comprehensive Cardiac Center certification
2017	Pinnacle of Excellence Award for inpatient satisfaction from Press Ganey

	Growth and Financial Stability
1999	Jayhawk Primary Care expansion
2002	First fully automated medical laboratory
2006	Opened new $77-million Center for Advanced Heart Care
2007	Opened new $36-million Richard & Annette Bloch Cancer Care Pavilion
2008	Opened a state-of-the-art Comprehensive Spine Center

2011	New medical office building opened
2011	Addition of Kansas City Cancer Center expands cancer footprint
2012	Expanded the geographic footprint with opening of Indian Creek Campus
2015	Health system assumes operation of Marillac Psychiatric Hospital for children and adolescents
2017	Opened the $360-million Cambridge Tower with 11 operating rooms and an initial 92 beds
2017	Acquired Hays Medical Center and Pawnee Valley Community Hospital
2017	St. Francis Hospital, Topeka, joins the health system through partnership with Ardent Health Services
2018	Expanded the footprint of Indian Creek Campus
2018	Great Bend Regional Hospital joins the health system
2019	Strawberry Hill Campus, the expanded home for adult behavioral health, opens
2019	Proton therapy announced

	Critical Partnerships
2000	Became healthcare partner of Kansas Speedway
2007	Sprint Center partnership
2011	Became the healthcare partner of the Kansas City Royals
2012	Became the healthcare partner of the Kansas City Chiefs
2014	Launched the Kansas Heart and Stroke Collaborative
2019	Launched Kansas Team Health with KU Athletics

Staying Out of the Red

The Five-Star Guiding Formula infused the business model with a *Do the Right Thing* moral compass. Time would tell whether taking the high road could keep KU Health System from losing money—but that didn't take much time.

"Operating revenue has grown in the right direction every year," confirmed CFO and Senior Vice President Doug Gaston. "This has put us in a position to invest in capital improvements."

Revenue Rebound 1999-2020

	Total Revenues
FY 08	$668,692
FY 09	$750,499
FY 10	$805,049
FY 11	$869,206
FY 12	$1,062,181
FY 13	$1,163,337
FY 14	$1,320,250
FY 15	$1,514,836
FY 16	$1,734,972
FY 17	$2,234,552
FY 18	$2,379,832
FY 19	$2,723,129
FY 20	$2,836,337

The model produced measurable progress, even if the measurement tools have differed over the years.

"One of the strengths of the Five-Star Guiding Formula has been consistency," Tammy Peterman said. "We haven't changed the business model since we established it, yet what we're doing within each of the five strategic areas is a very dynamic process. I think that's been key—continuously reaching for higher levels of performance on a foundation that's solid."

LEADERSHIP LESSON:

We've sustained our Five-Star Guiding Formula as a business model since we established it. That part doesn't change, although what we're doing within each of the five strategic areas is a very dynamic continuous improvement process. That's been key—continuously reaching for higher levels of performance works if your foundation is solid.

Proof of Performance: Five-Star Outcomes

Five-Star Measure	Goal/Measure	Rationale	Sustained Performance	Current Performance
Service	Overall rating of care performance in the top 10%* of large hospitals across the country on the CMS HCAHPS Survey as measured by Press Ganey.	This goal keeps the system's focus on the patient and reinforces the commitment to national leadership in delivering an optimal patient experience.	Consistently at or above the top 10% of large hospitals since 2013.	FY20 results show performance at the 92nd percentile (higher is better) —better than 92% of hospitals in the database.
Quality	Risk-adjusted mortality index, as calculated by Vizient using their most current risk-adjustment models, in the top 15% of comprehensive academic medical centers.	A strong risk-adjusted mortality index reflects the effectiveness of the care systems in delivering high-quality, evidence-based care.	Since December 2006, fewer actual deaths than statistically projected and consistently rank among the best CAMCs according to Vizient.	Final FY20, performance achieved the 9th percentile (lower is better) —better than 91% of the 100 comprehensive academic medical centers.
People	Employee retention (overall, nursing, and first-year) compares favorably to national and local benchmarks.	A strong retention rate provides a real-time sense of staff commitment to the vision and culture of the organization and is reinforced by regular engagement surveying.	The first significant change in the turnover rate, a 10% reduction compared to 1998, took place in FY01. The rate continued to decline in subsequent years.	FY20 overall turnover is 24% better than the national average, nursing turnover is 41% better than the national average, and first-year turnover is 10% better than the national average.

Strategic Growth	Overall year-over-year increase in patient volumes, strong market share, and a strong case mix index (CMI) for those patients cared for across the system.	As the tertiary/quaternary provider of care for the region, a strong CMI indicates the most acutely ill patients are seeking care here, and increased volumes and market share affirm the health system as the provider of choice for the area.	Incremental increase for the first few years with more substantial growth beginning in FY03; market share for FY02 was 6.3%. Currently take care of patients from every state in the U.S. and many international locations.	COVID-19 impacted patient volumes across the country. While inpatient volumes for the KC metro fell 4.1% during FY20, the health system inpatient volumes fell by only 1.5%. Market share for FY19 reached 13.6%; and over 2 million outpatient visits/encounters took place in FY20.
Financial Sustainability	Net operating income remains in the positive and achieves/exceeds the budget to support ongoing need for capital investment.	Maintaining profitability ensures the ability to invest in needed capital to support high-quality patient care and access to care.	Achieved profitability and an "A" bond rating early in the history of the authority.	From the inception of the hospital authority through FY20, the health system has remained profitable, supporting over $1.97 billion in capital investment.

* Using percentiles ensures performance keeps pace or exceeds the improvement pace of other hospitals.

"We're not just looking at progress, but opportunities for improvement," Peterman emphasized. "It's so important to celebrate our achievements, but there will always be new insights, methods, and approaches. We're not just implementing best practices, we're developing them, too. There are ways to keep raising the bar.

"I've said this a lot—we can be proud, but never satisfied—because thinking this way makes achievement part of continuous improvement—not just the end goal," she adds.

LEADERSHIP LESSON:

It's important to celebrate achievements, but there will always be new and better ways to keep raising the bar. We're not just implementing best practices, we're developing them, too. When we say *we're proud but never satisfied*, we're making achievement part of continuous improvement—not just the end goal.

The Secret Sauce for Sustainability

In 2019, Vizient, the nation's leading healthcare service company, identified three hospitals in the U.S. that had sustained high performance on the annual quality and accountability study over the history of the process. KU Health System was one of them. Page and Peterman welcomed the Vizient team on campus that August to interview physicians; nursing leadership; staff members; executive leaders; leaders from various service departments; rapid response teams; staff from data and analytics, ambulatory care, and the cancer center; and members of the board of directors.

"It was an intense fact-finding mission. They wanted to know our 'secret sauce' for sustainability," Bob Page laughed.

The executive team would later learn that almost everyone interviewed repeated Peterman's mantra: *We can be proud but never satisfied.*

"By the end of the week, I think Vizient really heard that," Page affirmed. "It's not just something Tammy says…it's not a slogan we're trained to repeat—it's really what we're all about."

According to Vizient Group Senior Vice President Julie Cerese, what Vizient learned from its 2019 nationwide "Sustainers Study" was the best patient experience comes to life through a palpable intensity involving people, processes, decision-making, and board support.[5]

Consistent goals and reliable metrics were also common themes. For KU Health System, everything on the list is a component of its culture.

LEADERSHIP LESSON:

It's never one thing you do; it's the steps you take and keep taking every day that build the foundation for ongoing transformation.

HOW WE KNOW THAT

Sustaining Improvement

By 2006, KU Hospital was ranked 11th out of 81 academic medical centers in the country. We kept hearing what a remarkable achievement that was, considering we were ranked lowest in patient satisfaction in the nation in 1998 and didn't measure quality in the way we do now. When I look back, what really stands out to me is how we accomplished that before our Lean initiative, clinical integration, or IOS—even before we expanded from a hospital to a health system. This is how I know transformative actions are the key. It's never one thing you do; it's the steps you take and keep taking every day that lead to transformation.

We weren't knowingly applying John Kotter's principles for change,[6] but it's not surprising that our transformative actions have a basis in research on leadership and change management.

TUKHS Transformative Actions	Kotter's Countermeasures against Transformational Failure
Admit It	Establish a sense of urgency
Believe It	Form a powerful guiding coalition; Create and communicate a vision
Culture It	Institutionalize approaches
Magnetize It	Empower others to act on the vision
Question It	Empower others to act on the vision
Improve It	Consolidate improvements and produce still more change
Integrate It	Consolidate improvements and produce still more change
Advance It	
Celebrate It	Plan for and create short-term wins
Sustain It	

For us, transformation has also included actions that *advance it* and *sustain it* (no Kotter countermeasure). And we apply an overarching process with steps that build on each other like a pyramid to ensure a strong CI model that's effective and evergreen: the C2C Pyramid.

The C2C Pyramid has culture in its foundation. It advances through critical elements of organizational performance. The culmination of efforts always leads to celebration…**c**ulture to **c**elebration (C2C).

C2C Pyramid

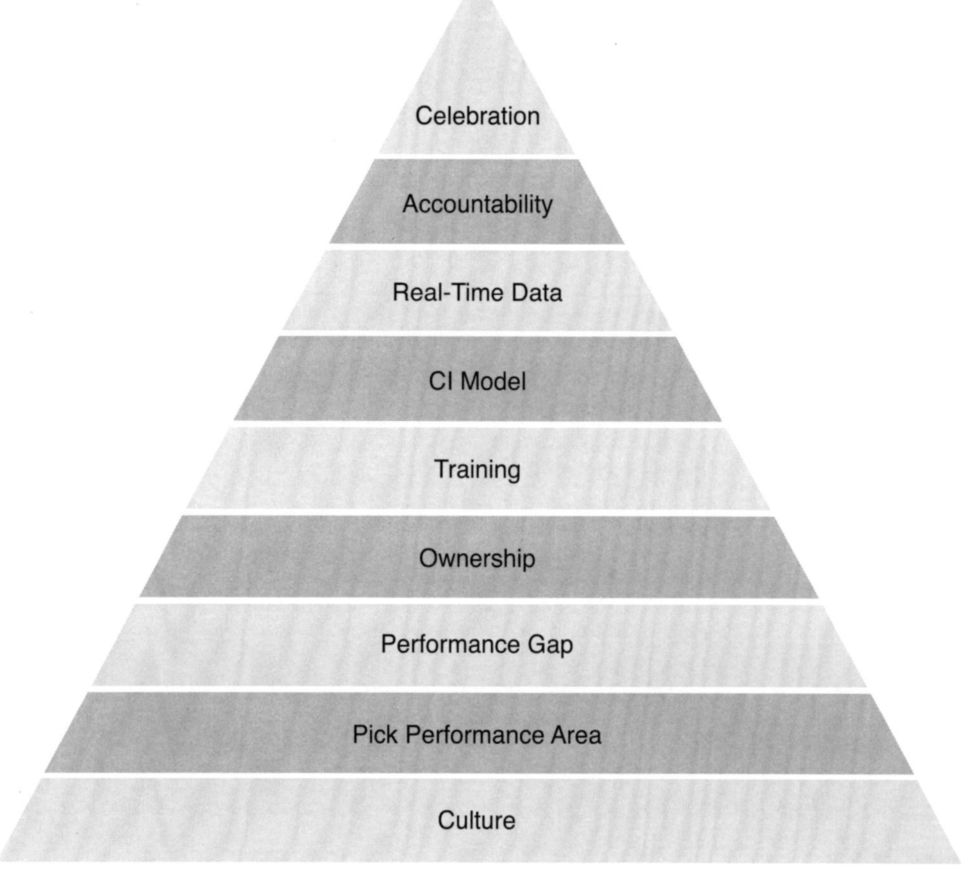

The *performance areas* are directly tied to organizational priorities. Once selected, current performance is compared to desired performance through external benchmarking to help identify the *performance gap*. The *owner* of the process selected for improvement works with internal resources to provide the necessary *training* to ensure the team is adept at the *continuous improvement model* chosen. As the improvement work progresses, *real-time data* is gathered to determine progress made and to assist in holding leaders *accountable* for improving performance. Once the goals are met or tangible improvement is made, *celebrations* occur to acknowledge progress and recognize the team for their efforts.

In the spirit of being "proud but never satisfied," the process then begins anew. The key to this method is a culture that supports and promotes continuous improvement—not just in words but in actions. Our job as leaders is to sustain this culture through our words and actions every day.
—Bob Page

Some Things Never Change

Huron healthcare consultant Chris Drummond believes the lessons of the past have endowed KU Health System with a resilient, agile culture that will help the organization avoid significant disruption in the future.

"I've actually met with the executive teams from 85 healthcare systems in the last 12 months, and a good share of those were academic medical centers," Drummond said. "After 25 years in this business, I have a really good feel for the culture of different AMCs out there. KU Health System is unique. They have more passion around the mission of the organization than any other organization I've worked with—and they're very protective of their culture."[7]

They've done a better job of sustaining change than other organizations I've worked with.

Drummond recalled the first time the Huron Consulting Group team worked on-site at KU Health System.

"We were given a scavenger-hunt checklist with ten things to do to get to know this organization's culture," he said. "It wasn't a rhetorical exercise—it was about direct engagement."

Protecting the culture doesn't mean resisting change.

"It's about making sure we're making choices that sustain our culture," Page explained. "We do pursue change proactively—but not for the sake of change. If we can see the potential, we're absolutely going to try a new approach that could help us improve our outcomes."

And from Chris Drummond's point of view, "They've done a better job of sustaining change than other organizations I've worked with."

HOW WE KNOW THAT

Sustaining What We Learned from the Pandemic

How could any of us have ever been prepared for a worldwide pandemic? I've never been more grateful or humbled by the quality and commitment of the people who work for this health system—and for the supportive community around us.

We discovered we could do things a lot more quickly than we thought we could when facing the novel coronavirus disease. Full implementation of our telehealth initiative was still in the project queue in the early spring of 2020 when the first COVID-19 cases came through our doors. In order to maintain social distancing and serve patients who were afraid to come here physically, we had to ramp that up swiftly.

Within 10 days, 2,500 Zoom licenses were issued so our doctors could do remote visits—1,086 in the first week and over 60,000 in the first 12 weeks. That brought approximately 70 percent cancellations per day down to under 30 percent. In fact, some days were down closer to 20 percent during the second week when we served 4,400 patients via telehealth. We set a goal of 2,500 telehealth visits every day by May.

Before we *had* to do it, we thought it would take up to a year and a half to do it. But when it became absolutely necessary, we had telehealth up and running in less than two weeks—that's a testimony to how agile our teams are.

Before we *had* to do it, we thought it would take up to a year and a half to do it. But when it became absolutely necessary, we had telehealth up and running in less than two weeks—that's a testimony to how agile our teams are.

We also remodeled our ambulance bay, creating 12 rooms where staff could take care of patients safely apart from other patients. That happened over one weekend—because it was the right thing to do.

Similarly, thanks to the philanthropic support to purchase an additional piece of testing equipment, we moved the locker rooms of the clinical labs and created the clinical space to house that equipment—also over the course of a weekend. By Monday, the equipment was ready for installation and quality testing/validation.

We started functioning at a speed that was possible only because agility was already built into this culture. We got creative in sourcing the supplies we knew would be needed to manage a large and sustained volume of COVID-19-positive patients.

We created an internal website—a kind of coronavirus-central—for employees and physicians to access up-to-the-minute information on hospital policy and status updates. We posted our "Take-10" daily videos from leadership to answer questions staff was asking, along with health tips for taking care of themselves as they took care of others.

Everything we did was an escalation of things we planned to do. We'd built capacity along the way, but we had to accelerate everything 1,000 percent.

In the midst of so much stress and anxiety and grief, we knew our own people and the community at large needed not only healthcare, but strength and leadership. We facilitated collaboration in many venues locally and across the state. Steve Stites, our

CMO, even brought CMOs from other hospitals into our daily Medical News Network briefings, and made our studio available to them. There have been opportunities for greater collegiality, and it's important to acknowledge that.

LEADERSHIP LESSON:

Look for the lessons in everything—even in, and especially in, a pandemic.

When we look for the lessons in everything—especially during a crisis—the benefits of what we've learned will stay with us, including:

- Technology enhancements such as the expansion of telehealth capabilities to 2,500 providers in less than two weeks and the installation of cutting-edge testing equipment to support timely COVID-19 testing for our staff and others across the community.
- Enhanced internal and external communication to ensure our staff, partners, and the community were receiving timely, fact-based, and actionable information. These include daily press briefings; weekly physician informational updates broadcast live; daily Take-10 updates for staff and physicians; and daily email updates for physicians, staff, and leaders.
- Increased connections across the region, state, country, and beyond. These include routine communication and collaboration with local municipalities, daily consultation with the Department of Health and Environment, and utilization of the Care Collaborative to ensure hospitals across the state have access to the most current science and technologies. We have been on calls with physicians in Wuhan and across the country to understand what approaches were most successful for keeping staff safe and helping patients survive.
- We have been the recipient of amazing community support, reinforcing the importance the community places on us. This included the donation of over $1 million in testing equipment and supplies to ensure adequate testing was available, thousands of meals for staff and physicians, and gifts of PPE for staff and patients.

Here's what I know—every day someone comes to us with a healthcare crisis that, for them, is every bit as unexpected and terrifying as COVID-19. Our job is to be prepared for all of that, every single day. The pandemic may have prompted or accelerated these steps, but they're improvements we will maintain.

Our belief is that everything we've learned, we can sustain. All of these improvements and more will stay with us going forward.
—Tammy Peterman

Although this COVID-19 pandemic has strained us all—ourselves personally and our institutions—TUKHS has taken on the challenge in very special ways. Yes, it has risen and expanded to take care of patients during the COVID-19 surge as it always has—tirelessly, efficiently, and in a caring manner. But what has set this health system apart is the leadership role it has assumed. By *not* waiting to be rescued by the federal government or the state, TUKHS built its own testing capacity, did community outreach for case discovery, and leveraged its academic and analytic capabilities to do what academic medical centers do best: educate and inform. The Morning Media Update is but one aspect of that. TUKHS has been a convener of many audiences—the public, caregivers, communities in the Kansas City metro region, and beyond.[8]
—Lee Norman, MD, Secretary of the Kansas Department of Health and Environment

The Power of Philanthropy

The funding mechanisms for an academic medical center are limited. There are dollars provided by the state (for TUKHS, state dollars are directed to the academic enterprise and not the health system), research grants, funds generated by the clinical enterprise, and philanthropy.

After years of underfunding and lack of capital investment before becoming a public authority, philanthropic support was essential for delivering on the commitment to improve the health of Kansans.

When Richard Bloch was admitted to the cardiac unit at KU Hospital in the early 1990s, he and his wife, Annette, first experienced what was special about this institution even then. The staff made numerous modifications to the space so the family could stay close at hand. Accommodations like that have long since been built into the physical setting at The University of Kansas Health System, but the Blochs never forgot the extraordinary responsiveness.

"We had such amazingly wonderful treatment," Annette said. "Everyone on the staff was pleasant the moment you walked in the door."

Richard and Annette had raised their family in Kansas City and were deeply committed to the community and to the mission and vision of its premier healthcare provider. So when Annette was diagnosed with breast cancer herself, "there was no question as to where I was going," she affirmed. The then-widow of the late co-founder of the H&R Block mega-accounting corporation, Annette "could have gone anywhere in the country and I chose to come here, which was a wonderful choice."[9]

In 2008, Annette Bloch announced the largest philanthropic gift to date for the University of Kansas Hospital—$20 million for the Richard and Annette Bloch Cancer Care Pavilion. Her endorsement sent a loud message to the philanthropic community in Kansas City.

As new initiatives to advance the health system's goals were identified, the philanthropic community engaged again and again. Other donations, including $1 million from the Burns & McDonnell Foundation, began to arrive. Significant contributions from the physicians themselves and cardiothoracic surgeon Dr. William "Bill" Reed and his wife, Mary, helped make the creation of the Center for Advanced Heart Care possible.

When plans were announced for Cambridge Tower, the goal of raising $100 million in charitable support was established. The campaign was led by former TUKHS Board Chair Greg Graves and his wife, Deanna. Annette Bloch was the first to step forward with a $10 million challenge grant. Others, including Cheryl Lockton Williams and Bill and Mary Reed, answered that call. The successful drive culminated in a way no one could have imagined.

In September 2018, a crowd gathered in the largest auditorium on campus for a special meeting to announce a $66-million gift—the largest ever in the history of the health system—from the Sunderland Foundation. Its purpose was to support the completion of the three remaining floors of the Cambridge Tower. Charlie Sunderland, former KU Hospital Authority board member and chair of its board quality committee, said, "We feel very comfortable making this grant, which will be used well to help a lot of people and improve the quality of lives for years to come."

Knowing the organization in the way the Sunderland family did, it was a resounding endorsement of progress made and progress to come.

The lesson in all of this is the importance of having a vision of what the health system wanted and needed to achieve, a culture that could turn that vision into a reality, and, ultimately, the deliverables showing the philanthropic community their contributions would achieve results.

And the philanthropic spirit that breathed life into the vision helped sustain the health system during the COVID-19 crisis.

In the first months of the 2020 COVID-19 crisis, over 800 donors contributed nearly $1.4 million—300 of these donors were grateful patients. Those donations included PPE, COVID-19 testing equipment, and much-needed supplies. One donation allowed TUKHS to purchase additional equipment to support testing in surrounding counties. And over 16,000 meals were contributed to staff in recognition of their long, stressful hours.

Back to the Future: What Will Tomorrow Look Like?

Although the pandemic changed the world in an unprecedented manner, the anticipation of change is not new at TUKHS. On any given day, Tammy Peterman, Bob Page, and the executive leadership team have considered what that day could look like ten years into the future.

Page pondered, "What will patients need from us? How will we continue to attract and retain the best people for this health system? What will the community and state need?"

Our mission is to provide the best possible healthcare in Kansas, the region, and the nation, and we are well poised to make that mission a reality. Just because you live west of Topeka doesn't mean you shouldn't have access to the very best care available. Whether it is cancer, heart, or many other service lines, we are capitalizing on collaboration and technology to ensure citizens across our state have access to the cutting-edge care and services provided by our nationally ranked health system.[10]
—Robba Moran, TUKHS Board Chair

For Peterman, "Ten years from now, we will have more hospitals in our system. We will have helped improve the health of Kansans, and we will have played a key role in redefining and implementing a sustainable healthcare delivery system across the state. That's our job and our role as an academic medical center.

"Most importantly, we will have maintained our core culture focused on high-quality, patient-centered care delivered by great people," Peterman assured. "We will have created a rock-solid foundation for advancing our mission and vision far into the future."

"And we will have applied the lessons we've learned from a pandemic," Page added.

LEADERSHIP LESSON:

We pinpoint five to ten years into the future as the starting point, then create a plan starting in the now to get us there. What will patients need from this health system then? How will we attract and retain the best people? We want to get the widest angle on the longest view to find the most viable answers.

Such *future-back* thinking is one of the new approaches to strategic planning for change.

"We want to get the widest angle on the longest view," Terry Rusconi explained. "There are things no one can see coming, especially since COVID-19. We don't think of what we do as business-as-usual, but as business-as-innovating-and-improving for the what-if and what-can-be. We have to plan accordingly."

> As physicians, we take an oath to care for patients. Every one of us was thinking of that even as the COVID-19 pandemic surfaced two competing themes: science and fear. Too often, fear frustrates science. Our medical staff confronted the fear and acted on science, allowing us to provide exceptional care and support to all patients across this health system. Our experience dealing with COVID-19 has reminded us who we really are, and we will carry that throughout our careers. I have no doubt what we have learned through this pandemic will positively inform and direct the way we care for patients for years to come.
> —Steve Stites

Anticipating future needs combines the future-back approach with on-going real-time progress toward identified stretch goals. Page and Peterman have numerous goals on the list:

- **Integrate the state.** As we have grown across the state, we have not yet fully integrated each of the locations into a holistic approach for clinical care and operations. We remain on different IT platforms and don't yet have consistent processes for supply chain and other critical systems. The comprehensive plan we are in the process of deploying will fully integrate all components of our existing system and establish the model for quickly incorporating additional organizations into the system.
- **Hurt no one—ever (zero harm).** We have not yet achieved zero harm across the health system, and this remains an essential commitment to our staff, our patients, and our communities. We have made great progress and have implemented some key approaches such as IOS. But as of today, we are not yet there, and we will continue with this work until we have achieved zero harm and know it can be sustained.
- **Become one.** We have seen significant impact since launching integration in 2016. Yet, there are so many additional opportunities to enhance collaboration across the

system, to standardize care and processes, and to create the best possible practice environment for our physician partners.

- **Improve the health of all Kansans.** Again, a lot of great work is taking place through the Care Collaborative and by bringing organizations into the system. However, we feel a great responsibility for ensuring every Kansan has access to the best possible care close to where they live. Included in this work will be strategic service line expansion, the expansion of telehealth, and work to recruit talented medical personnel to areas where needs exist.
- **Invest in our people.** Our staff and the culture they have helped enable and sustain have been the foundation on which our system has been built. We must continue to advance systems and processes that ensure we hire, onboard, support, and advance talented and committed staff who live out our culture in everything they do.
- **Ensure an inclusive environment.** Like many organizations, we are working to honor the diversity of our team, our patients, and our community. Starting at the senior leadership level, we are leading the efforts to understand, to improve, to measure success, and to build the best place to work for all staff, physicians, and patients.
- **Prepare for the next big challenge.** Our culture and infrastructure have taken on and effectively managed the COVID-19 pandemic so far. We know this will not be the last challenge our organization faces, so taking time to hardwire the lessons learned and identify approaches to address potential gaps in systems and processes will be important for future success.
- **Keep sharing what we've learned.** We are a health system that has benefitted from the lessons learned by other organizations as they have advanced their performance. We are also an organization called to share what we have learned. From the beginning, our focus has been on ensuring patients across our region, state, and country have access to the very best care and outcomes. One of the most important ways to make that happen is to share what we have learned through our journey—what worked, what didn't, and what we have identified as being foundational for success.

The Top Decile

Continuous improvement is a dynamic process even if the stated target never moves.

"When I talk to my colleagues across the country, I'm often surprised by how they set their performance targets," Page said. "Many are satisfied at the 50th percentile. One CEO of a nationally recognized, world-class facility told me they targeted the 75th percentile for patient satisfaction. I just shook my head. We do this very differently—maybe because we were once at the 5th percentile. What it took to transform this hospital from that low point in 1998 to the highest-percentile performance group in this country—in less than 10 years—is a culture that sustains our guiding formula."

At this health system, "Our goal is to be at the 90th percentile or better, or to be achieving stretch goals that will quickly get us to top decile performance," Tammy Peterman stated. "Unless we're in the top decile of performance for a metric—or exceeding those stretch goals—no one gets a green light for that measure of performance on our scorecard. Our goal is to be the best.

"Frankly, if you're not performing at that level, you're not consistently putting patients first, and that's what it's all about for us," Peterman added.

The *U.S. News & World Report* honor roll and Vizient's top-performing hospitals set the standard KU Health System holds itself accountable to "in order to provide world-class care," Page explained.

"We benchmark against the best," he added. "The regular comparative scorecards we receive from Vizient allow us to gauge our patient satisfaction and mortality numbers against the best comprehensive academic medical centers in the country. Going back to 2007 when Vizient was still the University HealthSystem Consortium, its Quality and Accountability Scorecard showed we were in the top decile of all those facilities. We were among the best of the best compared to them and have sustained that performance many years since."[11]

Peterman is quick to point out "the comparison isn't about competition. It's about getting better faster. We're thinking like people who function optimally in a continuous-improvement culture. If we're striving to do better today than we were doing yesterday, we have to be at the 90th percentile or higher, even as the performance level it takes to achieve that goal continues to increase."

LEADERSHIP LESSON:

We're thinking like people who function optimally in a continuous-improvement culture. If we're striving to do better today than we were doing yesterday, we have to be at the 90th percentile or higher, even as the performance level it takes to achieve that goal continues to increase.

The Green Carpet Story

At the top of the escalators off the main foyer, Greg Graves turns left and heads toward KU Health System's executive offices at the end of the long hallway. After 12 years on the TUKHS Board of Directors including two terms as chair, Graves has walked this stretch hundreds of times, and one thought always occurs to him.

"This hallway might just be the ugliest place in the entire hospital," he admits with a laugh.

In contrast to the Chihuly-style glass suspended near vaulted airy windows of the main entrance and sleek, art-curated newer facilities around campus, this inauspicious hallway features green indoor-outdoor carpeting halfway up unadorned white walls.

"There's a very good reason for that," Graves explains. "I hope it's not lost on the various visitors to the executive offices of this health system that Bob Page and Tammy Peterman won't be replacing that carpet until every other improvement goal has been met in this organization."[12]

Bob Page and Tammy Peterman won't be replacing that carpet until every other improvement goal has been met in this health system.

Guardians of the Culture

The unassuming surroundings fit the practical, steady administration of The University of Kansas Health System. Bob Page and Tammy Peterman, a CPA and nurse respectively, inspired by what could be, have blended their individual competencies as president/CEO and executive VP/COO/CNO and president of the Kansas City Division. For more than 20 years, the partnership has provided transformative but humble leadership. When it comes to accolades, both of them quickly widen the spotlight to their people.

“It’s not about the leader; it’s about the team of people,” Page insisted. “The leader’s job is to make sure you have the right team and make sure they have what they need to be successful, then let them do their job.”

Fundamentally, it should “plug and play” even as leaders and team members change.

“I think too many leaders think it’s all about them,” Page said. “Like the story of Lee Iacocca when he left Chrysler—the organization didn’t know what to do because it was all about Iacocca. I don’t want to diminish great leadership, but it needs to work like the Patriots when Brady was suspended for four games in New England. The Patriots didn’t miss a beat. The team had a system that works.”

LEADERSHIP LESSON:

The leader’s job is to make sure you have the right team, make sure they have what they need to be successful, then let them do really good work.

Peterman also resists grandstanding. After time spent providing direct patient care herself, that real-world experience informs everything about her approach.

“As I moved into roles of increasing responsibility as an executive, I had a lot to learn,” she affirmed. “But some of the most important skills I draw on every day were learned early on. The most important leadership skills come from experience, life, and continuously learning from others, like my dad. You bring those lessons with you when you’re the leader whose job is to sustain a culture in which the team can do great work.”

LEADERSHIP LESSON:
The most important leadership skills come from experience, life, and continuous learning. You bring those lessons with you when you're the leader whose job is to bring out the best in your team.

Page remembers well the lessons of his formative years at TUKHS.

"Too many leaders sit in their office thinking great thoughts but having no connection with their people and the work that happens on a daily basis," he said. "When I took over, I put on a housekeeping uniform one day and I went up and cleaned rooms. On another day, I worked in the emergency room and answered the phone. There was the day I went up and I just sat in the OR. I didn't work the schedule, but I watched the schedule work. It was just for learning."

Peterman thinks, "We've both been willing to acknowledge that leaders don't and can't know everything—we're both eager to grow, learning from one another and many others along the way."

Page agrees, "Leaders advance for a variety of reasons, but not because they know it all."

Leaders don't and can't know everything. They advance for a variety of reasons, but it's not because they know it all.

A Legacy Worth Upholding

When Page and Peterman calibrate plans for a sustainable future, "We want to ensure this institution is not only well maintained, but well positioned for continuous improvement," Peterman said. "Effective leadership is not just guiding a good, strong organization while you're there, but making sure the steps you took to accomplish that will be effective and replicable for years to come."

In the middle of Kansas, it's this extraordinary system. It's much more than the "little engine that could." It's really world-class on many dimensions. It's very successful, but what is unique about Kansas is that they were very successful and still wanted to be so much better.[13]
—Mike Rona

Succession planning is part of that process. "Like it or not, we're all aging every day," Page acknowledges. "Tammy and I think of ourselves as guardians of the culture. If we've built the right culture here, as long as we grow and advance leaders who believe in its values—who perpetuate and guard it with every decision they make—we've created something sustainable together."

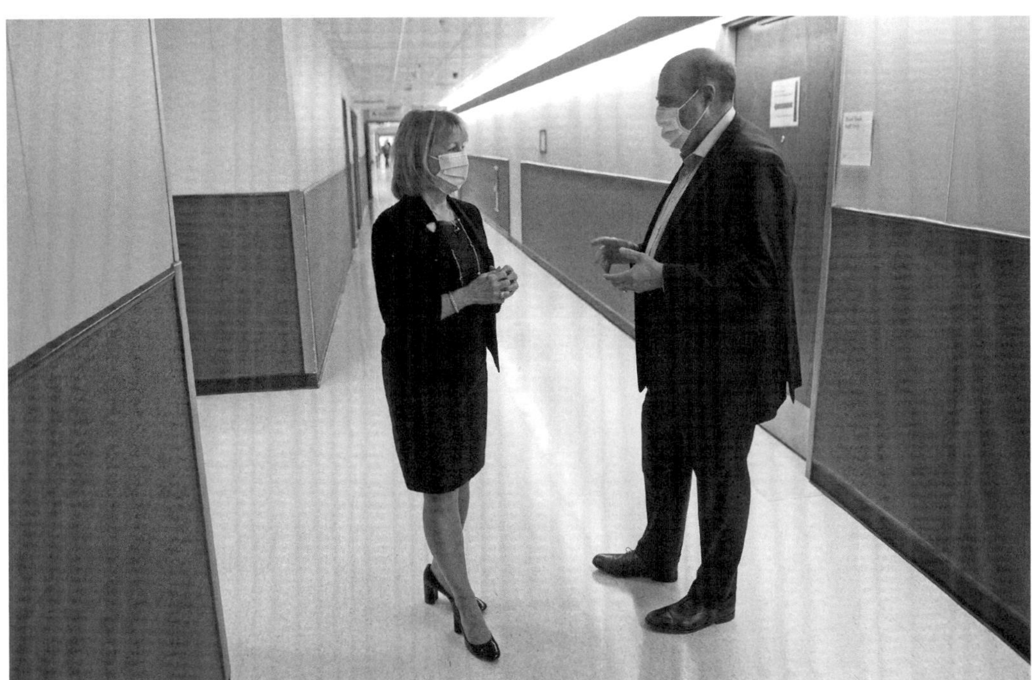

The green carpeted walls aren't what's remarkable. The leadership of Bob Page and Tammy Peterman is.

Ringing the Bell Together

Elizabeth Fuller was a frontline EMT finishing her paramedic license when the COVID-19 pandemic lockdown began in March 2020. Her job was indispensable, but as her colleagues dealt directly with the stress, anxiety, and exhaustion of the pandemic without her, Elizabeth watched from the sidelines.

More specifically, from inside the window in a room at KU Cancer Center.

When Elizabeth found a lump in her breast three months earlier, the 32-year-old mother of three was surprised to learn she was too young for a routine mammogram. The complicated, confusing process to get a referral then a definitive test at a local hospital took until mid-February.

With no family history of cancer, Elizabeth was shocked to learn she had stage 3 invasive ductal carcinoma. The diagnosis came with "no real information. There was nothing…just 'you have breast cancer.' It was a very scary experience," she recalled. "But everyone around us kept saying, 'You have to go to KU; they have the best cancer center.'"

So she did.

"It made a world of difference—to be in a teaching hospital with clinical trials and the wealth of information," Elizabeth said. She learned everything she needed to know about what she was going through from her new oncologist, Dr. Anne O'Dea, a medical breast oncologist at KU Cancer Center.

There were many options for treatment. "That was nice because having cancer during a pandemic is just one more thing that feels so out of control," Elizabeth said.

With her mom and husband, Steven, there for moral support, she got through her first three-hour chemo treatment. But a week later, absolutely no visitors were allowed due to pandemic restrictions. For the next six months, "I had to do all my treatments completely alone," she said. Without a loved one present to lend support and encouragement, Elizabeth's stress and anxiety intensified.

At one point, Elizabeth noticed another patient wearing a t-shirt that read *No One Fights Alone*. It was supposed to be inspiring, but, "I just cried," she said, feeling her isolation even more acutely. The nurses "were wonderful, but they're not my family. It's not the same."

But that t-shirt wisdom would prove itself.

Steven Fuller worked with the nurses to get his wife a room with a window overlooking the parking lot. On the strip of grass below, family and friends gathered every Friday so Elizabeth could see their faces while chatting with them on her cell phone or waving from her room during treatment.

Finally, it was her last day.

"On the first day of chemo, I heard someone ring the bell," she said. "I didn't know much about it. I thought it was silly and awkward." But as time went on, the grueling mental and physical side effects took their toll. Hearing that bell reminded Elizabeth that people do survive cancer… there could be an end to this. It helped her keep fighting.

Steven, her kids, mom, and so many friends had been experiencing this in their own right. "We all went through this together. I mean it might have been my fight, but they were with me through the whole thing," Elizabeth said. Everyone needed closure. "I told my husband I wanted my family to be with me when it was my turn to ring that bell," she said.

That was going to be problematic with the COVID lockdown still in place. Ringing the bell on the last day of chemo is a tradition at many hospitals, and a Zoom or Skyped-in audience is a go-to "virtual" compromise, but the KU Cancer Center staff surprised the Fullers with a unique solution.

"They literally built up a huge brass bell on the lawn of the cancer center, and I got to go down there and ring it," Elizabeth beamed.

Amidst an appropriately distanced entourage of nurses, her oncologist, friends, and family, she celebrated that moment surrounded by her people. Steven Fuller said, "For the kids, too, they got to see everyone lifting up their mom."

It was powerful. Elizabeth felt "it helped my four-year-old grasp that I don't have to keep doing this."

While there would be radiation and hormone treatments ahead, "just the joy of that moment... being able to say 'I did it' was remarkable," Elizabeth said. "Not everyone gets to have an end to chemo. Being able to say 'I'm done' is a huge victory."

Life beyond cancer felt possible again to Elizabeth Fuller; her vocation of helping others was enriched by what she'd experienced. "The cool thing about being an EMT and paramedic is we deal with cancer patients," Elizabeth said. "I'm excited to bring that knowledge back to work—not just as a provider but because I have the empathy of someone who's been through it."[14]

The large brass bell that was customized for Elizabeth remains at the ready for others. It will bear witness to the stories and mark the celebrations of many more who come to the place Dr. Simeon Bell envisioned as "the best medical care available anywhere" back in 1905.

More than 115 years later, that vision has never been clearer to the dedicated people who proudly embody the culture of The University of Kansas Health System.

Epilogue

Well, we did it. After being asked for the past ten years to write this book, it's finally done. And who would have ever thought we would finish the book during the biggest health crisis of our lifetimes: the COVID-19 pandemic!

As we write this epilogue, despite battling the greatest financial challenges we have faced since becoming a public authority, we ended the year with a positive bottom line from operations.

And, true to our culture, we achieved those results without laying off or furloughing any hospital or medical staff. In fact, we committed to securing our staff knowing we would come out of the crisis stronger than we were before.

What lessons do we hope you'll find helpful? And what have we learned that will benefit us as we prepare for our new world post-pandemic? Here's the list:

1. **It's all about culture.** Borrowing from Peter Drucker's famous phrase, we presented "Without Culture, Strategy Doesn't Even Get Invited to Lunch" at a national conference. The takeaway: Cultural transformation starts at the top. It can't be delegated.
2. **People are the most important asset in any organization.** For us, the combination of competence and humility are bedrocks of our system. And it isn't about any one person. It's always about the team.
3. **The patient always comes first.** The key is to ask yourself what your core business is. For us, our core business is patient care. When the patient is at the center of every decision we make, we make better decisions.

4. **It's about outcomes, not processes.** Improving processes is important, but only if it improves outcomes. And improving outcomes requires organizational honesty and integrity in evaluating data. Without data transparency, improving outcomes is impossible.
5. **Never underestimate the power of storytelling and celebration.** It is paramount for the team to know we, as leaders, know their stories and share their stories. We also need to celebrate victories, no matter how small. Celebrations create momentum, which accelerates success.
6. **Be proud but never satisfied.** Once leaders become satisfied, progress stalls and performance slips. As the old saying implies, there is danger in reading your own press clippings.

At The University of Kansas Health System, we have made great progress over the past 21 years. In fact, we have accomplished things no one thought were ever possible.

But there are two legs to our journey to becoming the best health system in the country. First, we have to get there…then we have to stay there.

To date, we haven't yet reached either of those destinations. By our standards, we never will. It's not only about being the best; it's about continuously improving…as we get better, the bar just gets higher. This is what drives us every day.

—Bob Page
—Tammy Peterman

Endnotes

Foreword

1. U.S. News & World Report. *U.S. News & World Report Rankings & Ratings*. U.S. News & World Report L.P. 2020-21.

Chapter 1: Admit It

1. Carey, Raymond G., Robert C. Lloyd. *Measuring Quality Improvement in Healthcare: A guide to Statistical Process Control Applications*. Milwaukee: Quality Press, 1995.
2. IBID
3. Toby, Bruce. Interview with Leeanne Seaver. Oral History Interview. January 2018.
4. The University of Kansas Healthcare System. *The University of Kansas Hospital Health Information Management Data*. The University of Kansas Healthcare System. 1995-2020.
5. Press Ganey. Means & Ranks. 1997.
6. Thompson, Irene. Interview with Arthur Daemmrich. Oral History Interview. October 2014.
7. Daemmrich, Arthur. *The University of Kansas Hospital (A): Structure, Strategy, and Organizational Culture*. Unpublished Case Study. Last Modified September 2015.
8. IBID.
9. Jackson, Jon. Interview with Arthur Daemmrich. Oral History Interview. September 2014.
10. Glasrud, Scott. Interview with Arthur Daemmrich. Oral History Interview. September 2014.
11. Thompson, Irene. Interview with Arthur Daemmrich. Oral History Interview. October 2014.
12. Wilk, Kenny. Interview with Leeanne Seaver. Oral History Interview. October 2017.

13. Lash Group. *Executive Summary: The New for Ownership/Governance Change at KU Hospital.* AmerisourceBergen Corporation, 1997. 6-7.
14. Graves, Governor Bill. Interview with Leeanne Seaver. Oral History Interview. October 2017.
15. Page, Bob. Interview with Leeanne Seaver. Oral History Interview. October 2017.
16. Rusconi, Terry. Interview with Leeanne Seaver. Oral History Interview. September 2017.
17. Ross, Frank. Interview with Arthur Daemmrich. Oral History Interviews. September 2014
18. Honse, Bob. Interview with Leeanne Seaver. Oral History Interview. September 2017.
19. U.S. News & World Report. *U.S. News & World Report Rankings & Ratings.* U.S. News & World Report L.P. 2019.
20. IBID
21. Vizient. UHC Quality & Accountability Study. Vizient. 2005-2020
22. U.S. News & World Report. *U.S. News & World Report Rankings & Ratings.* U.S. News & World Report L.P. 2019.
23. IBID
24. National Cancer Institute. *NCI-Designated Cancer Centers.* U.S. Department of Health and Human Services. July 2020.
25. The Hospital Consumer Assessment of Healthcare Providers and Systems (HCAHPS). *HCAHPS: Patients' Perspectives of Care Survey.* U.S. Centers for Medicare & Medicaid Services. 2018.
26. CardioVascular Learning Network. *University of Kansas Health System First to Achieve Joint Commission Comprehensive Cardiac Center Certification.* Journal of Invasive Cardiology. July 20, 2017.
27. The University of Kansas Healthcare System. *The University of Kansas Hospital Health Information Management Data.* The University of Kansas Healthcare System. 1995-2020.
28. Lieberman, Lily, Andrew Vaupel. *Forbes names Garmin, 14 other KC-area firms as 'best employers' in Kansas.* Kansas City Business Journal. June 25, 2019.
29. Rona, Mike. Interview with Leeanne Seaver. October 2019.
30. Pingleton, Susan. Interview with Arthur Daemmrich. Oral History Interviews. October 2014.

Chapter 2: Believe It

1. Thompson, Irene. Interview with Arthur Daemmrich. Oral History Interview. October 2014.
2. IBID
3. The University of Kansas Healthcare System. *The University of Kansas Hospital Health Information Management Data.* The University of Kansas Healthcare System. 1995-2020.
4. Jackson, Jon. Interview with Arthur Daemmrich. Oral History Interview. September 2014.
5. Daemmrich, Arthur. *The University of Kansas Hospital (A): Structure, Strategy, and Organizational Culture.* Unpublished Case Study. Last Modified September 2015.
6. Kansas Statutes, Chapter 76, State Institutions and Agencies; Article 33, University of Kansas Hospital Authority, 3304.
7. Glasrud, Scott. Interview with Arthur Daemmrich. Oral History Interview. September 2014.
8. Girod, Doug. Interview with Leeanne Seaver. Oral History Interview. December 2017.
9. The University of Kansas Healthcare System. *The University of Kansas Hospital Health Information Management Data.* The University of Kansas Healthcare System. 1998-2020.
10. Gaston, Doug. Interview with Leeanne Seaver. Oral History Interview. July 2019.

Chapter 3: Culture It

1. Nawalanic, Gregory. Interview with Leeanne Seaver. Oral History Interview. April 2020.
2. Peterman, Tammy. Interview with Leeanne Seaver. Oral History Interview. June 2020.
3. Page, Bob. Interview with Leeanne Seaver. Oral History Interview. November 2017.
4. Peterman, Tammy. Interview with Leeanne Seaver. Oral History Interview. November 2017.
5. Miller, Paula. Interview with Leeanne Seaver. Oral History Interview. September 2017.
6. McGuirk, Joseph. Interview with Leeanne Seaver. Oral History Interview. August 2018.

7. IBID
8. Mohta, Namita Seth, Stephen Swensen. *Organizational Culture Is the Key to Better Health Care.* NEJM Catalyst. April 2019.
9. Carlton, Liz. Interview with Leeanne Seaver. Oral history Interview. November 2018.
10. Uhlig, Mark. Interview with Leeanne Seaver. Oral History Interview. January 2018.

Chapter 4: Magnetize It

1. Peterman, Tammy. Interview with Leeanne Seaver. Oral History Interview. September 2017.
2. Jackson, Jon. Interview with Arthur Daemmrich. Oral History Interview. September 2014.
3. Wolters Kluwer Health, Inc. "Workplace Empowerment and Magnet Hospital Characteristics: Making the Link," *Journal of Nursing Administration* 33, (2003) 410-422.
4. American Nurses Credentialing Centers. *Magnet Recognition Program: About Magnet.* American Nurses Association; American Nurses Credentialing Center; American Nurses Foundation. 2020.
5. Graystone, Rebecca. *National Magnet Nurse of the Year 2017 Award Winners.* HealthCom Media. January 18, 2018.
6. The University Kansas Health System. *Accreditations and Awards.* The University of Kansas Health System. 2020.
7. Walsh, Teresa. Interview with Leeanne Seaver. Oral History Interviews. September 2017.
8. Pickering, Casey. Interview with Leeanne Seaver. Oral History interviews. June 2018.
9. The University of Kansas Health System. *FY18 RRT Database.* June 2018.
10. IBID
11. Setter, Robin. Interview with Leeanne Seaver. Oral History Interview. April 2018.
12. IBID

Chapter 5: Question It

1. Trzeciak, Stephen. "Knowledge@Wharton," *Wharton Business Radio.* Sirius XM, Philadelphia, PA: Channel 132, Aug 6, 2018.
2. Centers for Disease Control and Prevention (CDC). *Healthcare-Associated Infections (HAI) Data Index.* U.S. Department of Health & Human Services. 2018.

3. The University of Kansas Health System. *National product recall started with our alert RNs.* 24/7 TUKHS intranet. July 2018.
4. MedTech Intelligence Staff. *Becton Dickinson Recalls More than 151 Million Alaris Infusion Sets.* Innovative Publishing C. LLC. July 19, 2019.
5. Drummond, Chris. Interview with Leeanne Seaver. Oral History Interviews. October 2020.
6. Zidel, Thomas G. *Lean Done Right.* Chicago: Health Administration Press. 2012.
7. Ruder, Chris. Interview with Leeanne Seaver. Oral History Interviews. August 2020.
8. The Inpatient Operating System (IOS). Defect Reports. University of Kansas Health System. 2020.
9. IBID
10. Mahnke, Miki. Interview with Leeanne Seaver. Oral History Interviews. February 2020.
11. IBID, Ruder.
12. Gartner, Amanda. Interview with Leeanne Seaver. Oral History Interviews. August 2019.

Chapter 6: Improve It

1. Press Ganey. Means & Ranks. 2007-2020.
2. Daemmrich, Arthur. *The University of Kansas Hospital (A): Structure, Strategy, and Organizational Culture.* Unpublished Case Study. Last Modified September 2015.
3. The Institute for Healthcare Improvement. Rapid Cycle Improvement Model. 1999.
4. The University of Kansas Hospital. Key Statistics Report. June 2018.
5. Page, Bob. Interview with Leeanne Seaver. Oral History Interview. February 2018.
6. Huron Healthcare. Case Study. December 2014.
7. Press Ganey. Means & Ranks. 2006.
8. Miller, Jon, Jaime Villafuete, Mike Wroblewski. *Creating a Kaizen Culture.* McGraw Hill Education. 2014.
9. Zidel, Thomas G. *Lean Done Right*, 115. Chicago: Health Administration Press. 2012.
10. Press Ganey. Means & Ranks. 2020.
11. Lasack, Collette. Interview with Leeanne Seaver. Oral History Interview. September 2019.
12. Wright, Jeff. Interview with Leeanne Seaver. Oral History Interview. September 2019.

13. Industry Week. Manufacturing Performance Institute Census of Manufacturers Report. Endeavour Business Media, LLC. 2007.

Chapter 7: Integrate It

1. American Hospital Association (AHA). Member Pulse Survey. AHA News. March 9, 1998.
2. Association of Academic Health Centers (AAHC). *AAHC Research & Analysis: Key Perspectives for AHC Leaders*. AAHC. 2014.
3. Collins, Christopher. Interview with Leeanne Seaver. Oral History Interview. December 2019.
4. Collins, Christopher T., Michael F. Rotondo, Steven W. Stites. *Leadership & Management: The Inevitable Call for Integrated Academic Health Systems*. Becker's Health Review. April 26, 2019.
5. Pingleton, Susan. Interview with Arthur Daemmrich. Oral History Interview. October 2014.
6. Stites, Steven. Interview with Leeanne Seaver. Oral History Interviews. December 2017.
7. Marting, William. Interview with Leanne Seaver. Oral History Interviews. November 2020.
8. Benson, Kirk. Interview with Leeanne Seaver. Oral History Interviews. June 2019.
9. Collins, Chris. Interview with Leeanne Seaver. December 2019.
10. Toby, Bruce. Interview with Leeanne Seaver. Oral History Interviews. January 2018.
11. Sale, Keith. Interview with Leeanne Seaver. Oral History Interviews. February 2020.
12. Long, Shawn. Interview with Leanne Seaver. Oral History Interviews. February 2018.
13. Barnes, Austin. *25th anniversary: Roasterie founder Danny O'Neill recalls humble start with just 'nickels and pickles.'* Startland News. September 7, 2018.

Chapter 8: Advance It

1. Brown, Chris. Video Diary. The University of Kansas Healthcare System (TUKHS). 2020.
2. US Fed News. *USPTO Issues Trademark*. Medical News Network. November 12, 2017.
3. Meltwater. National Media Monitoring Analytics Report of March 31-May 18, 2020. Meltwater. March 31-May 18, 2020.

4. Brandt, Tom. Interview with Leeanne Seaver. Oral History Interview. May 1, 2020.
5. Thompson, Irene. Interview with Arthur Daemmrich. Oral History Interview. October 2014.
6. IBID
7. Pierce, Lynelle, Stepheny Berry, James Howard, Kahdi Udobi, Cris Pritchard, Niaman Nazir, Michael Moncure. "Daily Spontaneous Awakening Trial in the Sedated Mechanically Ventilated Patient in the Surgical ICU," *Critical Care Medicine* 42, no.12 (December 2014) A1556-A1557.
8. The University of Kansas Health System. *Data Management System.* The University of Kansas Health System. 1995-2020.
9. Kumer, Sean. Interview with Leeanne Seaver. Oral History Interview. October 2019.
10. Peterman, Tammy. Interview with Leeanne Seaver. Oral History Interview. March 2018.
11. Butler, Tori. Interview with Leeanne Seaver. Oral History Interview. April 2018.
12. Jones, Matt. Interview with Leeanne Seaver. Oral History Interview. April 2018.
13. Eickmeyer, Sarah. Interview with Leeanne Seaver. Oral History Interview. January 2020.
14. Wild, David. Interview with Leeanne Seaver. Oral History Interview. November 2019.
15. Moser, Bob, Jodi Schmidt. Interview with Leeanne Seaver. Oral History Interview. April 2020.
16. The University of Kansas Health System. *Data Management System.* The University of Kansas Health System. 2016-2019.
17. Moser, Bob. Interview with Leeanne Seaver. Oral History Interview. March 19, 2020.
18. Dykstra, Brenda. Interview with Leeanne Seaver. Oral History Interview. May 2020.
19. Roeder, Amy. *Zip code better predictor of health than genetic code.* The President and Fellows of Harvard College. August 4, 2014.

Chapter 9: Celebrate It

1. Carlton, Liz. Interview with Leeanne Seaver. Oral History Interview. June 2018.
2. "New Immunotherapy Called CAR T Saves Young Mom With Cancer." Medical Miracles. *Megyn Kelly Today.* NBC. Feb. 22, 2018. Television.
3. Simonds, Gary, Wayne Sotile. *Thriving in Healthcare: A Positive Approach to Reclaim Balance and Avoid Burnout in Your Busy Life.* Pensacola: Studer Group, LLC (2019).
4. Siers, Gigi. Interview with Leeanne Seaver. Oral History Interview. April 2018.

5. Studer, Quint. *Hardwiring Excellence.* Pensacola: Studer Group, LLC (2003).
6. Edwards, Katy. Letter to Page & Peterman. March 2019.

Chapter 10: Sustain It

1. Bailey, Cara, Pat Hagan, Howard Jeffries, Joan Wellman. *Leading the Lean Healthcare Journey: Driving Culture Change to Increase Value.* Boca Raton: CRC Press, LLC. 2017.
2. Banty, Karl, Christopher Collins, Dan Harrison. *Are Integrated Academic Health Systems Better?* ECG Management Consultations. November 9, 2015.
3. Pingleton, Susan. Interview with Arthur Daemmrich. Oral History Interview. October 2014.
4. Marso, Andy. *KU Hospital was barely breathing 20 years ago. Here's why it's thriving now.* The Kansas City Star. November 3, 2017.
5. Cerese, Julie, David Levine. *Quality and Accountability Continuing the Quest for Excellence.* Microsoft PowerPoint Presentation. Vizient. January 2020.
6. Kotter, John P. "Leading Change: Why Transformation Efforts Fail," *Competitive Strategy.* 1995.
7. Drummond, Chris. Interview with Leeanne Seaver. Oral History Interview. January 2018.
8. Norman, Lee. Interview with Leeanne Seaver. Oral History Interview. October 2020.
9. Bloch, Annette. Interview with Leeanne Seaver. Oral History Interview. September 2017.
10. Moran, Robba. Interview with Leeanne Seaver. Oral History Interview. October 2020.
11. Page, Bob. Interview with Leeanne Seaver. Oral History Interview. December 2017.
12. Graves, Greg. Interview with Leeanne Seaver. Oral History Interview. May 2020.
13. Rona, Mike. Interview with Leeanne Seaver. Oral History Interview. October 2019.
14. Plake, Sarah. KSHB News. *Mother overcomes battle with cancer, rings in end of chemo with friends, family.* Scripps Local Media. August 14, 2020.

About the Authors

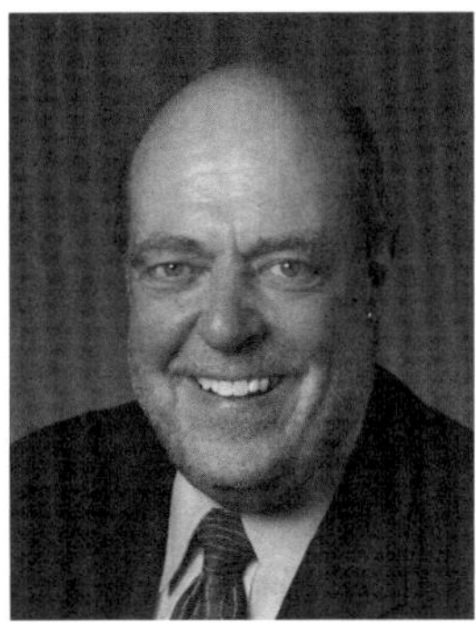

Bob Page has spent 24 years in executive leadership roles within The University of Kansas Hospital/Health System, a nationally recognized comprehensive academic medical center located in America's heartland. In July 2007, he was selected by The University of Kansas Hospital Authority Board to be president and CEO, a role that has grown as the organization became clinically integrated and expanded its commitment to patient care across the state.

Page has also worked to stabilize the healthcare environment across Kansas, a state with a widely dispersed population, the largest number of at-risk critical access hospitals identified as essential to their communities, and disaggregated resources to support optimal patient care and outcomes. Under his leadership, the health system committed itself to improving the health of Kansans through innovative collaborations with nearly 70 hospitals across the state, resulting in improvement in the use of evidence-based practice and patient outcomes.

The organization Page joined in 1996 was at risk of closure due to poor performance and financial insecurity. Throughout his tenure, he has relied on a simple formula, consistently grounded in a culture focused on the patient and the staff. That strategy and the foundation it established has resulted in quality recognized at a national level by both Vizient and *U.S. News & World Report*, high levels of staff engagement, top decile patient satisfaction, the completion of a five-year process to clinically integrate the medical staff and the health system, historic levels of capital investment, and significant growth.

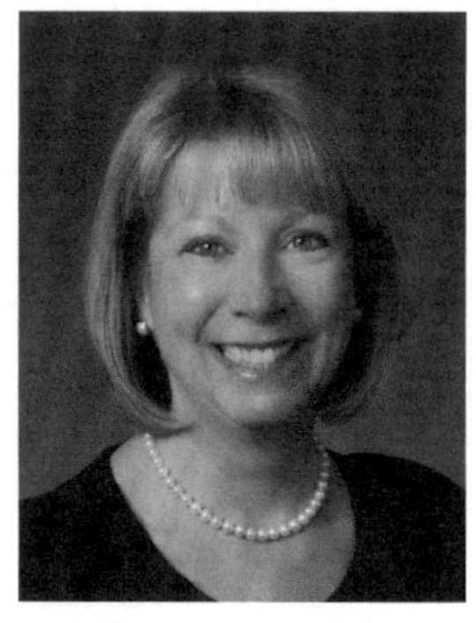

Tammy Peterman began her career as a bedside nurse at The University of Kansas Hospital after graduating from The University of Kansas School of Nursing. Since that time, she has served in a wide variety of nursing and hospital leadership roles. In 2001, she was appointed chief nursing officer for The University of Kansas Hospital. In 2007, Tammy added the titles of executive vice president and chief operating officer of the hospital. On July 1, 2018, Peterman became the executive vice president, chief operating officer, and chief nursing officer for the health system and president of the Kansas City Division.

Partnering with staff from across the organization, Peterman has championed initiatives focused on creating and sustaining a patient-centered culture capable of providing care and outcomes worthy of national recognition. This work has been grounded in staff engagement, the creation of a healthy work environment, effective onboarding and orientation, improved patient safety and patient outcomes, and strong interprofessional relationships.

Under her leadership, The University of Kansas Hospital/Health System has achieved many significant milestones, including designation as the first Kansas-based Magnet institution in 2006, with re-designation in 2011 and 2016. The hospital/health system has been recognized for fourteen consecutive years on *U.S. News & World Report's* Best Hospitals list, eleven years as the best hospital in Kansas City, and nine years as the best hospital in Kansas. The hospital has also been recognized as one of the high-performing comprehensive academic medical centers by Vizient's Quality and Accountability Study nine times, as of 2020.

In 2016, Tammy Peterman was inducted as a fellow into the American Academy of Nursing.

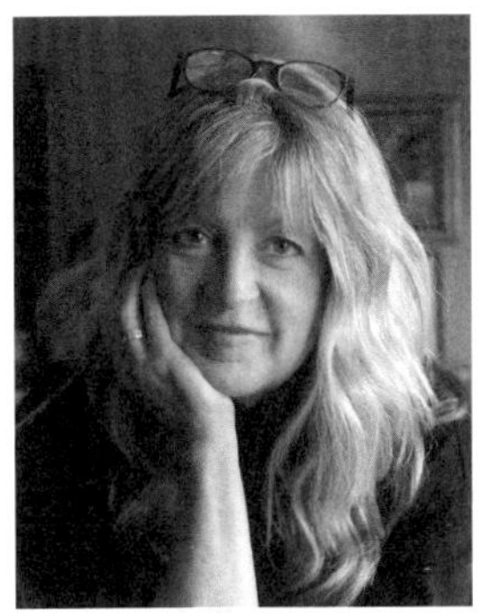

Leeanne Seaver is a cross-genre writer, editor, and blogger who's written/ghostwritten numerous books and magazine articles on healthcare and wellness. A member of the Authors Guild, Seaver's work ranges from business to biography, training to travel. She's been featured in *Mother Earth News*, *Redbook*, *Reader's Digest, Living Wellness Kansas City*, and is a contributor to the Medical News Network.

After a career in broadcasting and non-profit executive leadership, Seaver now writes full-time. She holds a master's in mass communication from the University of Denver, a bachelor's in English from Graceland University, and has attended the Iowa Writers' Workshop. See www.seavercreative.com.

Huron Learning Solutions

As the healthcare industry continues to transform, leaders and staff are being asked to do more with less, all while evolving their skills for a new reality. From embracing data-driven decision-making to understanding consumer needs to building their own resilience, the skills employees and organizations need to succeed in the future have changed.

Organizations must ensure their employees have access to comprehensive, relevant training and professional development that enables best-in-class performance, growth, and innovation.

From virtual, on-demand learning to customized, organization-wide coaching, Huron provides online and in-person training to meet your needs.

Speaking

Huron speakers are sought after for their ability to motivate diverse audiences, provide practical strategies on healthcare's most complex issues, and deliver field-tested solutions for immediate improvement.

From online executive training to large-association learning and development programs, our experts deliver the perfect balance of inspiration and education for every audience.

Online Learning

The online learning platform offers convenient and engaging education courses for employees at all levels, delivered virtually, on demand, and accessible from anywhere. Designed to promote individual, department, and organizational priorities, our education training provides the foundation to make goals more achievable than ever.

Conferences

Address change head-on with innovative solutions and inspired leadership at a Huron conference. Our events feature keynote speakers delivering industry-leading perspectives, as well as opportunities to network with other healthcare leaders. After attending an in-person or virtual conference, you will leave with practical tools and tactics to turn your challenges into opportunities. Continuing education credits are available for most events.

Huron Books

Develop the skills needed to deliver results across organizations with Huron's purpose-driven books. Authors provide insights for every healthcare leader, ranging from leadership development, patient and employee engagement, and more.

Learn More

To learn more, visit https://www.huronconsultinggroup.com/expertise/organizational-transformation-healthcare/learning-development.